Neuroscience Research Progress

# Astrocytes

# Structure, Functions and Role in Disease

# NEUROSCIENCE RESEARCH PROGRESS

Additional books in this series can be found on Nova's website under the Series tab.

Additional e-books in this series can be found on Nova's website under the e-book tab.

# NEUROLOGY - LABORATORY AND CLINICAL RESEARCH DEVELOPMENTS

Additional books in this series can be found on Nova's website under the Series tab.

Additional e-books in this series can be found on Nova's website under the e-book tab.

NEUROSCIENCE RESEARCH PROGRESS

# ASTROCYTES

# STRUCTURE, FUNCTIONS AND ROLE IN DISEASE

OSCAR GONZÁLEZ-PÉREZ
EDITOR

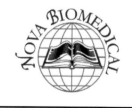

Nova Science Publishers, Inc.
*New York*

Copyright © 2012 by Nova Science Publishers, Inc.

**All rights reserved.** No part of this book may be reproduced, stored in a retrieval system or transmitted in any form or by any means: electronic, electrostatic, magnetic, tape, mechanical photocopying, recording or otherwise without the written permission of the Publisher.

For permission to use material from this book please contact us:
Telephone 631-231-7269; Fax 631-231-8175
Web Site: http://www.novapublishers.com

### NOTICE TO THE READER

The Publisher has taken reasonable care in the preparation of this book, but makes no expressed or implied warranty of any kind and assumes no responsibility for any errors or omissions. No liability is assumed for incidental or consequential damages in connection with or arising out of information contained in this book. The Publisher shall not be liable for any special, consequential, or exemplary damages resulting, in whole or in part, from the readers' use of, or reliance upon, this material. Any parts of this book based on government reports are so indicated and copyright is claimed for those parts to the extent applicable to compilations of such works.

Independent verification should be sought for any data, advice or recommendations contained in this book. In addition, no responsibility is assumed by the publisher for any injury and/or damage to persons or property arising from any methods, products, instructions, ideas or otherwise contained in this publication.

This publication is designed to provide accurate and authoritative information with regard to the subject matter covered herein. It is sold with the clear understanding that the Publisher is not engaged in rendering legal or any other professional services. If legal or any other expert assistance is required, the services of a competent person should be sought. FROM A DECLARATION OF PARTICIPANTS JOINTLY ADOPTED BY A COMMITTEE OF THE AMERICAN BAR ASSOCIATION AND A COMMITTEE OF PUBLISHERS.

Additional color graphics may be available in the e-book version of this book.

**Library of Congress Cataloging-in-Publication Data**

Library of Congress Control Number: 2012935715

ISBN: 978-1-62081-558-8

*Published by Nova Science Publishers, Inc. ✝ New York*

*To My Dear Beloved Ones*

*Elizabeth, Oscarín and Daniel*

# Contents

| | | |
|---|---|---|
| **Preface** | | ix |
| **Chapter I** | Role of Drug-Metabolizing Enzymes in Astroglial Function<br>*Amruthesh C. Shivachar, Dakota Jackson, and Shere Paris* | 1 |
| **Chapter II** | Astrocytic Potassium Channels in Central Nervous System Disorders<br>*Miroslava Anderova and Helena Pivonkova* | 17 |
| **Chapter III** | The Phosphoinositides Signal Transduction Pathway in Astrocytes<br>*Vincenza Rita Lo Vasco* | 37 |
| **Chapter IV** | Astrocytes as Neural Stem Cells in the Adult Brain<br>*Oscar Gonzalez-Perez* | 53 |
| **Chapter V** | Ultrastructural Characteristics of Astrocytic Neural Stem Cells in the Adult Brain<br>*Irene Sanchez-Vera, Arantxa Cebrian-Silla, M. Salome Sirerol-Piquer, and Jose Manuel Garcia-Verdugo* | 65 |
| **Chapter VI** | Aging, Environmental Enrichment, Object Recognition and Astrocyte Plasticity in Dentate Gyrus<br>*Daniel Guerreiro Diniz, César Augusto Raiol Foro, Marcia Consentino Kronka Sosthenes, João Bento Torres, Pedro Fernando da Costa Vasconcelos, Cristovam Wanderley, and Picanço Diniz* | 91 |
| **Chapter VII** | Role of Astrocytes in Viral Infections<br>*Cecilia Bender, Jesica Frik, and Ricardo M. Gómez* | 109 |
| **Chapter VIII** | Astrocyte Dysfunction in Megalencephalic Leukoencephalopathy with Subcortical Cysts<br>*Raúl Estévez* | 125 |
| **Index** | | 145 |

# Preface

The cellular composition of the adult brain comprises five major well-identified cell populations: neurons, astrocytes, oligodendrocytes, NG2-expressing cells and microglia cells. Astrocytes, commonly known as *astroglia*, are the most abundant cell type into the brain. Astroglial cells greatly outnumber neurons, approximately 10:1 and occupy up to 50% of the volume of the brain. Remarkably, astrocytes are the only cerebral cells that contain glycogen (the main energy storage molecule) and are thoroughly distributed into the brain including white and gray matter. Few decades ago, it was believed that astrocytes were inert cells that merely provided support or served as the putty to hold neurons together. Nevertheless, increasing evidence indicates that this was a misconception. In fact, astrocytes are the most important brain cell population for preserving tissue homeostasis and the main metabolic support for neurons by providing them with lactate. Some additional astrocytic functions include: neurotransmitter uptake and release, a blood–brain-barrier component, regulation of ion concentration in the extracellular space, modulation of synaptic transmission and plasticity, cerebral regulation of blood flow, nervous system repair, myelinating regulation, toxicity depuration and neuroprotection. Therefore, astrocytes are emerging as vital cells for cerebral functions and growing evidence indicates that they play a bigger role in the etiology of many brain disorders than previously thought.

This book summarizes the latest discoveries regarding the main roles of astrocytes in physiological and pathological circumstances. All chapters were written by world-wide-recognized experts in their respective fields. The authors have made their best to present all these information in an easy-to-understand language, which will benefit to a wide variety of readers, from undergraduate students to postdoctoral fellows or scientific colleagues from many disciplines. This book comprises the following eight chapters:

Chapter I - is an excellent analysis of the role of astrocytes in drugs metabolism. Therein, Shivachar et al., explain that astrocytes are capable of producing key metabolic intermediates of polyunsaturated fatty acid arachidonic acid, mainly by cyclooxygenase, lipoxygenase and cytochrome P450 epoxygenase pathways. They also discuss how epoxygenase pathways produce epoxide metabolites in astrocytes, which provide neuroprotection under both physiological and pathological conditions. The authors also propose that selective inhibitors of epoxide hydroxylase could be promising therapeutic drugs for the treatment of stroke. However, they warn that ubiquitous inhibitors activate alternative pathways for the metabolic conversion of reactive epoxides, which otherwise may make adduct by binding to proteins and nucleic acids. Consequently, they may cause an accumulation of defective proteins and mutated genes, leading to cancer and other conditions. Thus, further studies are required to fully establish the consequences of inhibitors of epoxide hydroxylase.

Chapter II - One of the key functions of astrocytes is to maintain $K^+$ homeostasis in the brain during neuronal activity, a process called potassium spatial buffering, in which astrocytic $K^+$ conductances play an important role. Potassium spatial buffering relays on the expression of inward-rectifier $K^+$ (Kir) channels. Anderova and Pivonkova present a very interesting chapter that summarizes current knowledge about the expression and functioning of Kir channels in astrocytes and also explain the role of aquaporins and connexins in brain disorders. The authors explicate how the expression and functioning of astrocytic Kir channels are seriously affected in acute and chronic pathological conditions, such as ischemia or epilepsy. In particular, the reduced Kir4.1 channel expression or Kir4.1 channel mislocations promote astrocytic depolarizations, which decrease their ability to clear excess of extracellular glutamate that contribute to neural damage. In summary, Anderova's chapter highlights the importance of astrocytic potassium channels in the maintenance of brain homeostasis and the role of them in the pathogenesis of some brain disorders.

Chapter III - The phospholipase C enzymatic family and the phosphoinositide signaling system are crucial for molecule transductions from plasma membrane to cell nucleus. This system appears to be involved in a number of neuronal and glial functions. In this chapter, Lo Vasco comprehensively describes the role of inositol lipid cycle in astrocyte activation during neurodegenerative processes. Herein, she shows recent evidence indicating that up- or down-regulation of different phospholipase-C isoforms contribute to astrocyte reactivity, cerebral inflammation and tumor progression. Therefore, this chapter is strongly recommended for neurobiologists interested in lipid metabolism in the brain tissue.

Chapter IV - In the adult mammalian brain, *bona fide* neural stem cells were discovered in the subventricular zone (SVZ), lining the lateral wall of the lateral ventricles of the brain. In this proliferative niche resides a subpopulation of glial cells that show immunoreactivity and ultrastructural characteristics, which allow identifying them as astrocytes. This subpopulation of SVZ astrocytes displays stem-cell-like features both *in vivo* and *in vitro*. The progeny of astrocytic progenitors are neuroblasts and oligodendrocyte precursors, which differentiate into mature interneurons and myelinating oligodendrocytes. Throughout life, these new-born cells populate the olfactory bulb and the white matter, respectively. Gonzalez-Perez's chapter summarizes current evidence that demonstrated the astrocytic nature of adult neural stem cells. Therein, he also describes the cellular composition and organization of SVZ progenitors and, reviews some of their molecular and genetic characteristics.

Chapter V - During embryonic development of the brain, neuroepithelial cells from the primordial ventricular zone transform into radial glial cells. These cells give rise to neurons and glia during brain development. In the postnatal brain, radial-glial-like cells are observed and during adulthood at least in two brain areas: the SVZ at lateral walls of the lateral ventricles, and the subgranular zone (SGZ) in the dentate gyrus at the hippocampus. Professor Garcia-Verdugo is the neuroscientist who for the first time described in detail the ultrastructural characteristic of astrocytic neural stem cells resident in the SVZ and the SGZ. In this outstanding chapter, the pioneer author and co-workers provide a unique, meticulous and complete description of the ultrastructural characteristic of astrocytic neural stem cells (and their progeny) in the germinal areas of rodent, primate and human brain. Therefore, this chapter is a mandatory reference for all professionals interested in studying adult neural stem cells in the SVZ and the SGZ.

Chapter VI - Astrocytes have been recently related to hippocampal-dependent tasks, such as episodic-like and spatial memory. Diniz and coworkers show data clarifying the role of astrocytes in object recognition tasks and cognitive performance. Interestingly, the morphological changes and regional distribution of astrocytes within the hippocampus appear to be dependent of both aging and enriched environments. The authors hypothesize these differential findings can be due to aging and housing environment. Both of these conditions target different subpopulations of hippocampal astrocytes; consequently, cells in the polymorphic and granular layer in the dentate gyrus show different proliferation rates.

Chapter VII - A neurotropic virus is a small infectious agent that is capable of infecting neural cells, or which does so preferentially. Such viruses evade the immune response and are able to infect astrocytes. Since astrocytes play a crucial role in cerebral homeostasis, viral infection in glial cells may alter such functions leading to serious neural damages and/or neurological complications. Interestingly, astrocytes also express class II major histocompatibility complex antigens, but their function is still not fully elucidated. Activated astrocytes express toll-like receptors crucial for the induction of innate immune responses, including the secretion of chemokines or cytokines in response to virus agents. In their chapter, Bender and co-workers explicate in plain words the role of astrocytes in immune response and neuroinflammation during viral infection.

Chapter VIII - Oligodendroglial cells provide a functional segmentation of the axolemma by producing myelin, which electrically insulates axons in the central nervous system. A fundamental function of astrocytes consists in modulating the myelination process of oligodendrocytes. Mutations in astrocytic-expressed genes are associated with leukodystrophies, a group of neurological disorders characterized by imperfect growth or development of the myelin sheath. Estevez explains the role of astrocytes in myelin homeostasis and describes the pathophysiology of megalencephalic leukoencephalopathy, which is interestingly characterized by astrocytic dysfunction. This chapter will be very interesting for those professionals interested in studying the myelination process in the central nervous system.

On behalf of the authors and my-self, I hope that readers find in this book a very useful compendium for their academic and research activities about the structure, function and role in disease of astrocytes. The editor expresses his gratitude to the people of *Nova Science Publishers* involved in this book production. I am particularly grateful to Dr. Arturo Alvarez-Buylla at the University of California at San Francisco and Dr. Jose M Garcia-Verdugo at the University of Valencia, as exceptional sources of insights and academic guidance on neuroscience research. Finally, I would like to express a great appreciation and gratitude to all my colleagues and mentors over the years. They are too many to list here, but I want them to know my gratitude. Recent collaborators include Alfredo Quiñones-Hinojosa, Rocio E. Gonzalez-Castañeda, Sonia Luquin, Alma Y. Galvez-Contreras, Norma Moy-Lopez, Jorge Guzman-Muniz, Veronica Lopez-Virgen, Tania Campos-Ordoñes, Jimena Rocha-Espejel, Lucia Alvarez-Palazuelos, Jorge Collas, Fernando Jauregui, Oscar Chavez-Casillas, Fernando Gutierrez and many others. I thank you all guys for your personal support, hard work, scientific contributions and invaluable ideas.

In: Astrocytes
Editor: Oscar González-Pérez

ISBN: 978-1-62081-558-8
© 2012 Nova Science Publishers, Inc.

*Chapter I*

# Role of Drug-Metabolizing Enzymes in Astroglial Function

*Amruthesh C. Shivachar*[*],
*Dakota Jackson*[#], *and Shere Paris*[#]
Department of Pharmaceutical Sciences, College of Pharmacy and Health Sciences,
Texas Southern University, Houston, Texas, US

## Abstract

Astrocytes are the principal glial cell type in the central nervous system (CNS). These cells are often regarded as supportive cells of the brain, performing mainly, neurotransmitters uptake, energy homoeostasis, neurotrophic factor release, and blood-brain barrier maintenance. Our own and other studies have produced a wealth of information suggesting that astrocytes are capable of producing key metabolic intermediates of polyunsaturated fatty acid arachidonic acid, mainly by cyclooxygenase, lipoxygenase and cytochrome P450 epoxygenase pathways. The latter pathway produces epoxide metabolites which protect astroglial, neuronal, and vascular networks in a concerted manner and preserve CNS function in health and disease state. Furthermore, inhibitors of metabolic degradation of these glioprotective epoxides by a soluble epoxide hydrolase have been shown to be novel therapeutic targets for maintaining neuronal health in ischemic injury. This book chapter summarizes recent advances in (1) astrocytes structure and function, (2) astrocytes drug metabolizing enzymes and (3) astrocytes drug metabolizing enzymes as putative targets for therapyin normal astrocyte physiology as well as pathological conditions.

---

[*] Address for correspondence: Amruthesh C. Shivachar, PhD; Associate Professor, Department of Pharmaceutical Sciences; Texas Southern University; 3100 Cleburne Avenue, Houston, TX 77004, USA; Tel: 713-313-1896; Fax: 713-313-4219; E-mail: shivachar_ac@tsu.edu.
[#] Graduate students who equally contributed in the literature search for this article.

**Keywords:** Astrocytes; Epoxyeicosatrienoicacids; epoxide hydrolase inhibitors; cytochrome P450 epoxygenase; microsomal epoxide hydrolase; soluble epoxide hydrolase

# Introduction

The brain is an assembly of two major cell types, neurons and glial cells. Glial cells are subdivided into different types with different functions: oligodendrocytes, microglial cells, ependymal cells and astrocytes. The astrocytes, commonly called as astroglia, are the most abundant glial cell type accounting for up to 30% of the brain's volume (Hertz et al 1998). In the brain, astrocytes are found distributed in both white and grey matter with slight differences in their morphology: more processes-bearing in the former and flat sheet-like in the grey matter (Somjen 1988). The flat sheet-like structures surround the synapses and send out numerous processes which ensheath some neuronal axons and impinge on small blood vessels as end-feet (Beck et al 1984; Hertz et al. 1998). These physical connections with neurons on one side and vascular cells on the other make astrocytes a versatile cell type capable of regulating neurotransmitter homeostasis, and blood-brain barrier functions.

Over the past two decades, a virtual revolution has occurred in our understanding of the physiology of astrocytes and of their interaction with neurons in the normal brain (reviewed by Takano et al. 2009; Kimelberg and Nedergaard 2010). Astrocytes actively propagate $Ca^{++}$ signals to neighboring neurons to modulate their synaptic activity (Thrane et al. 2011). Likewise, astrocytes communicate with neurons through glutamate and ATP/adenosine (Peng et al. 2009). Astrocytes also have recently been implicated in the local control of blood flow (Iadecola and Nedergaard 2007). Additionally, astrocytes are capable of metabolizing endogenous and exogenous chemicals, including neurotransmitters, fatty acids and sterols as well as environmental lipid-soluble chemicals which readily cross the blood-brain barrier. Astrocytes are known to express a wide variety of phase I and phase II drug metabolizing enzymes including cytochrome P450 enzymes, epoxide hydrolases and glucoronidases. Cytochrome P450 (CYP, P450) is the collective term for a superfamily of heme-containing membrane proteins responsible for the metabolism of approximately 70 - 80 % of clinically used drugs. Besides the liver and other peripheral organs, several CYP isoforms are expressed in glial cells and neurons of the brain (Meyer et al. 2007). This book chapter summarizes recent advances in (1) astrocytes structure and function, (2) astrocytes drug-metabolizing enzymes and (3) astrocytes drug- metabolizing enzyme as targets for therapy.

## Astrocytes Structure and Function

### Astrocytes Structure

In the healthy brain, astrocytes have been broadly classified into two main subtypes, *protoplasmic* and *fibrous* on the basis of differences in their cellular morphologies and anatomical locations. Protoplasmic astrocytes appear as star-shaped throughout the grey matter and often possess short, highly branched processes. In contrast fibrous astrocytes are found throughout the brain's white matter and exhibit long fiber-like processes. The neuroanatomical studies indicate that both subtypes make physical contact with blood vessels, but modern electron microscopic studies reveal that processes of protoplasmic astrocytes ensheath synapses and those of fibrous astrocytes are in physical contact with nodes of Ranvier and that both types of astrocytes form gap junctions between distal processes of neighboring astrocytes (Peters et al. 1991). While these observations are interesting, studies from others and our labs show astrocytes change their morphology under different culture conditions and in the absence of neurons or neuronal conditioned medium. Pure cultures of astrocytes either from rat brain (Figure 1, *panels* A, C and D) or from normal human brain (Figure 1, *panel* B) often show a "flat" sheet-like surface with smooth irregular amoeboid edges (Figure 1A and B). The same cultures undergo morphological changes upon addition of chemicals such as dibutyrylcAMP (Figure 1C) or addition of neuronal conditioned medium (Figure 1D), suggesting the involvement of neuronal derived factors responsible for their protoplasmic and fibrous morphology (Gegleshvilietal 1996; Hertz et al1998; ACS unpublished data, see Figure 1). These morphological attributes appear to be chemical rather than anatomical.

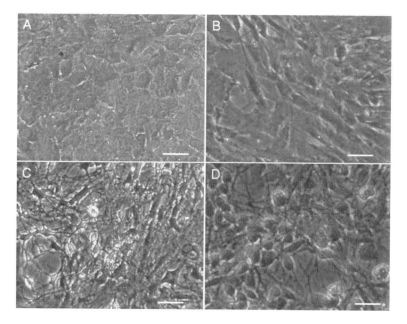

Figure 1. Representative phase contrast photomicrographs showing rat cortical astrocytes (panels A, C, D) untreated (panel A), treated for 5 days with dibutyryl-cAMP (250microM; panel C),or treated 5 days with neuronal conditioned medium (panel D) and normal human astrocytes (panel B) at 20x magnification. Neuronal conditioned medium was a cell-free nutrient medium obtained from highly enriched neuronal cultures and diluted with glial feed 1:1 ratio as described (Gegelashvilli et al. 1996). Scale bar: 100 μm.

Both astrocytes subtypes can be identified immunohistochemically by their ability to express the cytoskeletal protein glial fibrillary acidic protein (GFAP). GFAP is one of a family of intermediate filament proteins similar to vimentin, nestin and other that serve cytoarchitectural functions (Pekny and Pekna 2004). There are different isoforms and splice variants of GFAP, including α, β, γ, δ, and κ all of which may be expressed in healthy and pathological conditions, but their roles are only beginning to be understood (Andreiuolo et al 2009; Blechingberg et al 2005). However, it is important to note that GFAP expression is not exclusive to protoplasmic or fibrous astrocytes. Recent studies show that GFAP is expressed by other cell types within the brain (Bachoo et al. 2004) as well as outside of the brain (Bush et al. 1998; Ruhl 2005). Nonetheless, GFAP expression can be regarded as a sensitive and reliable marker for identifying the "astrogliosis" wherein activated astrocytes accumulate in response to brain pathological conditions and injury (Eng et al 2000; Faulkner et al 2004). Other molecular markers such as glutamine synthetase and $S100\beta$ have been used (Goncalves et al 2008; Norenberg 1979), but these molecules are not entirely specific for astrocytes.

## Astrocytes Function

Unlike neurons, astrocytes do not "fire" or propogate action potentials, even though they express potassium and sodium channels and evoke inward currents (Nedergaardet al.2003). However, astrocytes play an active role regulating the physiological functions of neighboring neurons and blood vascular cells through increases in intracellular calcium $(Ca^{++})_i$ concentration (Charles et al. 1991; Cornell-Bell et al. 1990). A large body of evidence show that increases in $(Ca^{++})_i$ as intrinsic oscillations triggered by transmitters or other extracellular stimulants propagates the message between astrocytes-astrocytes and astrocytes-neurons (Halassa et al. 2007; Nedergaard et al. 2003; Perea et al. 2009; Shigetomi la. 2003; Voltera et al. 2005 ) thus enabling astrocytes to play a direct role in synaptic transmission. Astrocytes also communicate with neighboring astrocytes through gap-junctions in normal and pathological conditions of brain (Nedergaardetal. 2003; Seifert et al. 2006). Astrocytes have been shown to play a role in brain development, in maintaining energy, ionic, pH, and transmitter homeostasis, and blood-brain barrier (Brown and Ransom 2007; Sattler and Rothstein 2006; Seifert et al 2006).

Astrocytes are known to fight against pathological conditions through astrogliosis, where they make a "scar" tissue at or near the impacted brain region and protect the neurons from the deleterious effects of locally produced toxicants, and thus forming a principal defensive mechanism (see reviews by Escortin and Bonvento 2008 and Sofroniew and Vinters 2010 and the references therein).

The intrinsic capacity of astrocytes to react to brain pathological conditions as a defensive mechanism makes them a potential therapeutic target to treat brain diseases. The development of defense mechanism in astrocytes may involve activation of several key mediators such as proteins, receptors and drug-metabolizing enzymes for the successful inactivation of neurotoxicants accumulated in the injured brain region. These enzymes may detoxify neurotoxicants or produce neuroprotective endogenous products to protect neurons from injury. Emerging evidence suggests that astrocytes express some of these enzymes which belong to the cytochrome P450 family and other drug- metabolizing enzyme classes as reviewed in the preceding section in this book chapter.

## Astrocytes Drug -Metabolizing Enzymes

### Astrocytes Cytochrome P450

Although drug metabolism is traditionally thought of as a function of the liver, there is now evidence that drug-metabolizing enzymes are also located in extrahepatic tissues, including the brain, where they appear to have important functions.

The brain drug-metabolizing enzymes mainly belong to the superfamily of cytochrome P450 (CYP). Cytochrome P450 enzymes (CYPs) are phase-I enzymes that are involved in the oxidative activation or deactivation of both endogenous and exogenous compounds such as drugs, environmental toxins and dietary constituents. By convention, each CYP family member is designated by a number, each subfamily by a letter and each member of the subfamily by a second number (e.g., CYP2D6).

CYPs have been shown to play a role in the activation or inactivation of centrally acting drugs, in the metabolism of endogenous compounds, and in the generation of damaging toxic metabolites and/or oxygen stress (Miksys and Tyndole 2002).

Several CYP family members have been detected in the brain some of which are distributed unevenly among brain regions, and are found in neurons, glial cells and at the blood-brain barrier interface. They have been observed in mitochondrial membranes, in neuronal processes and in the plasma membrane, as well as in endoplasmic reticulum (Miksys and Tyndale 2002; 2004).

Brain CYPs are inducible by many common hepatic inducers, however many compounds affect liver and brain CYP expression differently, and some CYPs which are constitutively expressed in liver are inducible in brain. CYP induction is isozyme-, brain region-, cell-type- and inducer-specific (Table 1). While it is unlikely that brain CYPs contribute to overall clearance of xenobiotics, their punctate, region- and cell-specific expression suggests that CNS CYPs may create micro-environments in the brain with differing drug and metabolite levels. The sensitivity of brain CYPs to induction may vary from individual to individual in response to centrally acting drugs and neurotoxins, and in the metabolism of endogenous compounds.

**Table 1. Region- and cell-specific distribution and the substrates of cytochrome P450 2 family, subfamily and their members in rat and human brain**

| Family | Sub-family | Members | Brain regions | | Cellular distribution | Substrate | References |
| --- | --- | --- | --- | --- | --- | --- | --- |
| | | | Rat | Human | | | |
| CYP2 | CYP2B | CYP2B6 | | cerebellum | Astrocytes/ neurons | Xenobiotics | Miksys S, Tyndole RF 2004 |
| | CYP2C | CYP2C8 | | endothelium | Endothelial | Arachidonic acid | Michaelis et al. 2005 |
| | | CYP2C9 | | Endothelium | Endothelial | Arachidonic acid | Michaelis et al. 2005 |
| | | CYP2C11 | Cortex Hippo-campus | | Astrocytes Astrocytes | Arachidonic acid Arachidonic acid | Liu M, Alkayed NJ 2005 Yamaura et al. 2006 |
| | CYP2D | CYP2D6 | | Substantian-igra | Neurons | alcohol | Miksys S, Tyndole RF 2004 |
| | CYP2E | CYP2E1 | Frontal cortex | Frontal cortex | Pyramidal neurons | Ethanol | Miksys S, Tyndole RF 2004 |
| | CYP2J | CYP2J2 | | | Aortic endothelial | Arachidonic acid | Yang et al. 2001 |
| | | CYP2J3 | Trige-minal | | Neurons | Arachidonic acid | Iliff and Alkayed 2009 |
| | | CYP2J4 | Trige-minal | | Neurons | Arachidonicacid | Iliff and Alkayed 2009 |

As shown in Table 1, cytochrome 450 2 family enzymes have been detected in the brain (Miksys and Tyndale 2004). Of these, astrocytes express CYP2 family members belonging to CYP2B, and CYP2C subfamily in rat and human brain (Miksys and Tyndole 2004). In rat brain, the CYP2B subfamily member CYP2B6, metabolizes nicotine and is shown to be expressed primarily in neurons (Anandatheerthavarada et al.1990; Rosenbrock etal.2001; Volk et al.1995). In normal human brain, the CYP2B6 enzyme is expressed in both neurons and astrocytes, high levels are found in neurons of hippocampus and cerebellum of smoking alcoholics (Miksyset al.2003). Interestingly, these are the same regions that are known to suffer damage after long term alcohol abuse (Fadda and Rossetti 1998).

CYP2D subfamily enzymes metabolize a variety of centrally acting drugs, including opioids, neuroleptics, anti-depressants, beta-blockers, and endogenous neurochemicals (Zhanger et al. 2004). Ethanol administration is shown to increase the expression of CYP2D subfamily enzymes in rat brain (Warner and Gustafsson 1994). Among CYP2D subfamily, highest activity of CYP2D6 member is observed in purkinje cells of cerebellum in smoking alcoholics (Miksyset al.2002).

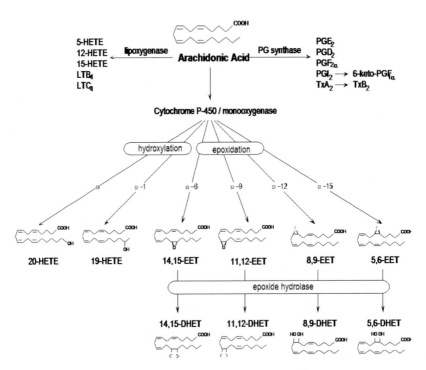

Figure 2. Diagram depicting arachidonic acid metabolism by cyclooxygenase, lipoxygenase and cytochrome p450 epoxygenase pathways in mouse brain (Amruthesh et al. 1992) and in rat hippocampal astrocytes (Amruthesh et al. 1993). Please note that cytocromeP450 metabolites were further metabolized into vic-diols by the soluble epoxide hydrolase activity in mouse brain slices and in rat cortical astrocytes.

CYP2E subfamily members metabolize many xenobiotics, including alcohol, acetaminophen, and tobacco-derived nitrosamines to carcinogenic metabolites (Leiber, 1999). The CYP2E1 is a subfamily enzyme metabolizes ethanol, and endogenous substrates such as arachidonic acid, and estrogenic metabolites (Leiber, 1999; Ohe et al. 2000). CYP2E1is expressed in high levels in human brain pyramidal neurons of frontal cortex, hippocampus, granular cells of dentate gyrus, and purkinje cells of cerebellum (Howard et al.2003).

Members of the CYP2C and CYP2J subfamily enzymes metabolize endogenous fatty acids, especially arachidonic acid, causing the hydroxylation and epoxidation of the so-called third branch of arachidonate cascade (see reviews,Capdevilla et al. 2002; McGiff et al.1999; Roman et al. 2002). The CYP2C and CYP2J subfamily members function as arachidonateepoxygenases and produce isoform-specific sets of regio- and stereo - isomericepoxyei-castrienoic acids (EETs). Our group has previously demonstrated dilation of cerebral arteioles by EETs, especially 5, 6-EET, using in vivo microscopy and the closed cranial window techniques in rabbits (Ellis et al.1990). We then, for the first time, demonstrated the biosynthesis of these vasoactive EETs in mouse brain slices (Amruthesh et al.1992). We subsequently demonstrated the cytochrome P450 epoxygenase pathway along with cyclooxygenase and lipoxygnease pathways (see Figure 2) in cultured rat brain cortical astrocytes (Amruthesh et al. 1993). In a further study, we demonstrated that exogenous EETs, especially 14, 15-EET uptake into astrocytes modulates PKC mediated phospholipases, suggesting possible activation of a kinase signaling pathway (Shivacharet al.1995) as shown in figure 3.

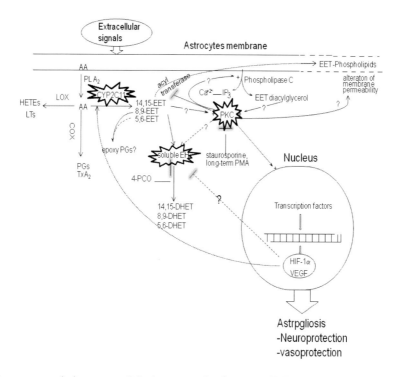

Figure 3. Diagram postulating some of the known and unknown cellular pathways for astroglial EETs production, incorporation, release, and metabolism in astrocytes in culture and possible regulation by a PKC-mediated signaling as previously described (Shivachar et al. 1995). The recent advances on the role of astrocytes in neuro- and vaso-protection against hypoxia-ischemic injury in the author's lab and in others lab is depicted as dotted lines. COX, cyclooxygenase; CYP2C11, cytochromeP450 epoxygenase; HIF-1α, hypoxia-induced factor-1α; LOX, lipoxygenase, PKC, protein kinase C; PLA$_2$, phospholipase A$_2$; VEGF, vascular endothelial growth factor.

Our above findings were later confirmed by another group which identified the cytochrome P450 epoxygenase responsible for the production of EETs in rat astrocytes as a member of the subfamily CYP2C11 (Alkayed et al.1996).

These authors have further shown that ischemic preconditioning induces upregulation of CYP2C11expression in brain causing reduction in infarct size after middle cerebral arterial occlusion in rats (Alkayed et al. 2002) and in astrocytes exposed to hypoxic condition (Liu and Alkayed, 2005). In the latter study, these authors have shown that hypoxia-induced astroglial tolerance is due to upregulation of CYP2C11 and possible production of EETs. Furthermore, the authors show that upregulation of CYP2C11 is dependent on activation of transcription factor, hypoxia-induced factor-1$\alpha$ (HIF1$\alpha$) as a cellular mechanism of tolerance to ischemia-like injury. The detection of CYP2C11 isoenzyme in normal astrocytes and its upregulation under hypoxic injury suggests a protective role for EETs in brain. However we have previously demonstrated that the EETs action is short-lived due to rapid metabolism by another Phase I drug metabolizing enzyme, epoxide hydrolase activity in *in vivo* rabbit brain (Ellis et al.1990), in mouse brain slices (Amruthesh et al. 1992), and in rat astrocytes (Amruthesh et al. 1993; Shivachar et al.1995). Thus it is very important to review the role of epoxide hydrolases in the regulation of astrocyte-derived EETs function separately in the preceding section.

## *Astrocyte Epoxide Hydrolases*

Epoxide hydrolases (EHs) are ubiquitously distributed in a wide variety of living organisms (see review by Newman etal. 2005 and the referencs therein). Although there are seven epoxide hydrolase subtypes known, this article focuses on two subtypes of epoxide hydrolases: microsomal (mEH), and soluble epoxide hydrolase (sEH). Like the CYPs, highest activity of epoxide hydrolases are detected in liver compared to that in the extra hepatic tissues, including the brain. Nonetheless, the brain epoxide hydrolases have been previously detected in the microsomal fractions (Ghersi-Egeaet al.1994; Schladt et al. 1986; Teissiere et al. 1998). We have demonstrated the epoxide hydrolase activity which rapidly converts astrocytes-derived EETs to their vic-diols, first in mice brain slices (Amruthesh et al.1992), and then in cultured astrocytes (Amruthesh et al.1993; Shivachar etal.1995). Our recent immunocytochemical double staining, and quantitative immunoblotting studies, combined with substrate-specific enzyme assays in the subcellular fractions, clearly show that astrocytes constitutively express both mEH and sEH (Rawal et al. 2009).

## *Microsomal Epoxide Hydrolase*

The mEH has been well studied and characterized (Arand et al. 1999; Craft et al. 1990; Friedberg et al.1994; Lacourciere et al.1993).The mEH protein is made of 455 amino acid residues corresponding to a 50 KDa protein (Jackson et al.1987). Unlike the brain CYPs, the brain mEH has been shown to be noninducible (Ghersi-Egea et al. 1987). The brain mEH is ubiquitously distributed in all the brain regions, but its cellular localization is mainly limited to glial cells rather than neuronal (Ghersi-Egeaet a. 1994; Teisser et al. 1998). These reports are in agreement with our own studies showing the mEH is constitutively expressed in astrocytes (Amruthesh et al.1993; Shivachar et al. 1995) and the protein and activities are distributed in the microsomal fractions of cultured astrocytes (Rawal et al.2009). The mEH is well recognized as a key enzyme in the metabolism of environmental contaminants.

Consistent with this fact, the majority of studies investigating the mEH substrate specificity have focused on its role in xenobiotic transformations. More recently, the molecular association of mEH with various cytochrome P450s was shown to affect the rate of substrate hydrolysis in vitro (Taura et al. 2002). Of the tested P450s, CYP2C11 appeared to play the greatest role in the association/activation of mEH. While well recognized as a critical enzyme in xenobiotic detoxification, the implication of mEH- dependent metabolism of endogenous lipid substrates is less well defined.

*Soluble Epoxide Hydrolase*

A number of EHs are found in the cytosol as soluble proteins within various cells. These include the "soluble EHs", the hepoxilin hydrolase, and the zinc-metalloprotein leukotriene A4 hydrolase. Although the soluble EHs (sEHs) enzymes are predominantly localized in the cytosol, sEHs have been found associated with microsomal fractions and peroxisomes (Newman et al. 2005). Each of these enzymes, except the leukotriene $A_4$ hydroxylase, is responsible for the hydrolysis of aliphatic epoxy fatty acids, including the EETs to their corresponding diols (Figure 2). The mammalian sEHs are homodimers of 62-kDa monomeric subunits (Beetham et al. 1993). Each monomer is comprised of two distinct structural domains, linked by a proline-rich peptide segment. The epoxide hydrolase activity resides in the 35-kDa C-terminal domain, which contains an α/ß-hydrolase fold structure. The other 25-kDa N-terminal domain contains a distinct α/ß fold topology with a functional phosphatase activity, with apparent specificity for fatty acid diol phosphates (Newman et al 2003). Like its microsomal counterpart, sEH is distributed in both in hepatic and extrahepatic tissues (Newman et al 2005). The brain sEH also appears to be widely distributed in most of the rodents and human brain regions (Marowsky et al. 2009; Sura et al 2008). However, there are discrepancies in the cellular distribution: few studies show exclusively neuronal localization (Liu and Alkayed 2005; Zhang et al. 2007) and others show that astrocytes also express sEH (Amruthesh et al. 1993; shivachar et al. 1995; Marowsky et al. 2009; Rawal et al.2009). These findings were further corroborated with immunoblotting and enzyme assay using specific substrates for sEH. Our findings were in agreement with previous immunohistological studies on the distribution of sEH in mouse brain (Marowsky et al. 2009) and human brain (Sura et al 2008) regions showing colocalization of sEH with GFAP expressing cells in the cerebral cortex region. However, surprisingly, another group (Zhang et al. 2007) could not detect any sEH staining in rat astrocytes but rather detected sEH expression only in the neurons.

## Astrocytes Drug-Metabolizing Enzymes as Targets for Therapy

After the monumental discovery of EETs by Capdevilla and his groups (1982), the cytochrome P450 epoxygenase pathway has evolved so much and helped us to understand the molecular mechanisms of various diseases related to cardiovascular and renal system. The EETs also may have numerous beneficial effects on the central nervous system, especially in ischemic stroke, inflammation and pain.

As the EETs are short-lived due to their metabolic conversion by brain sEH into corresponding vic-diols, sEH inhibitors may help augmenting the EET levels in the brain. It is presumed that vic-diols are less active compared to EETs, due to their higher solubility and increased renal excretion. Until we know more about these vic-diols, it is logical to think that by inhibiting sEH, one can increase the tissue levels of the beneficial EETs and that constitutes the pharmaceutical basis for the novel sEH inhibitor (sEHI) drug design. Another alternative approach would be to design drugs that are known to selectively induce the brain CYP2C11 subfamily members, thus increasing brain EETs levels. Since the EETs are primarily metabolized by the sEH, the pharmacological inhibition of this enzyme appears to be a feasible approach to increase EETs levels *in vivo*. However, the genetic variations among individuals associated with these enzymes may limit targeting this enzyme subfamily (See review: Iliff and Alkayed 2010).

The sEH is preferred because it specifically hydrolyzes the endogenously produced EETs, unlike other EHs which target the detoxification of xenobiotics and carcinogenic toxins (Newman et al.2005). Among the four regioisomers, 14,15-EET is the most preferred substrate, with a lowest $K_m$ and highest $Vmax$, and 5,6-EET is a poor substrate (Morisseau and Hammock 2005; Shivachar et al.1995). Because of the important contributions, mainly by Hammock and others to the sEH field, potent inhibitors to this enzyme are currently available and the first clinical trials in humans on sEH inhibition for heart diseases are underway.

Currently available sEH inhibitors are 1, 3-disubstituted ureas, amides and carbamates with $IC_{50}$ values in the low nanomolar range (Newman et al. 2003; 2005). These inhibitors specifically block the hydrolase activity without affecting the phosphatase catalytic domain (Newman et al. 2003). With these drugs, augmentation of EET levels has been demonstrated in vivo and in vitro studies, mainly for the intervention of vascular or inflammatory responses (Schmelzeretal. 2005; Smith et al.2005; Revermann et al.2009).

## Future Direction

sEHIs appear to be the next promising therapeutic drugs for the treatment of stroke for which there is no cure currently available. By selectively inhibiting only the sEH, these inhibitors can modulate both circulating and tissue EETs, and thus provide a broad range of protection against tissue injury/vascular dysfunction involved in the development of stroke. A note of caution is that by blocking the action of the ubiquitous enzyme sEH, sEHIs may activate an alternative pathway(s) for the metabolic conversion of these highly reactive epoxides, which otherwise, may make adducts by binding to proteins and nucleic acids.

This may cause the accumulation of defective proteins and mutated genes, leading to cancer and other conditions. In the same note, future studies should also focus on the effects of sEHIs on cancer, the second leading cause of human death worldwide. At present there is not much is known about the role of sEH on tumorogenesis or tumor metastasis and whether sEHIs have the potential to be future anticancer drugs.

# Conclusion

The astrocytes drug-metabolizing enzymes, mainly CYP2C11, its human homolog CYP 2C8, and sEH are the potential targets for future drug development to fight the debilitating brain diseases, including stroke, inflammation and pain. The beneficial effects of EETs can be amplified either by designing selective inducers of CYP2C11 (its human homolog CYP2C8) or by designing more potent active-site directed inhibitors of sEH. Because, EETs are potent vasodilators in the cerebral circulation, and protect astrocytes and neurons and endothelial cells by several known and unknown signaling mechanisms (see review by Iliff and Alkayed 2010), inhibition of EETs degradation will be beneficial. Moreover, sEHIs have therapeutic value against stroke since EETs are angiogenic, anti-inflammatory and antithrombotic in the brain circulation. Furthermore, genetic variants of CYP2C8 and sEH gene EPHX2 have been identified; they have not been linked with ischemic stroke risk (Marciante et al. 2008; Zhang et al.2008). Therefore, variant gene products properties should be taken into consideration in the future design of variant-specific inducers of CYP2C8 or inhibitors of sEH to increase the efficacy and potency of these novel drugs. Another potential tool for sEH inhibition is region-specific gene deletion rather than whole genomic knockout because sEH is an ubiquitous enzyme. The fact that a previous study (Zhang et al. 2008) showing sEH gene deletion only affected intra-ischemic cerebral blood flow but failed to protect neural cells, suggests additional underlying mechanisms requiring further research for the treatment of stroke, the most leading cause of disability and third leading cause of death worldwide.

# References

Alkayed N. J., Narayanan J., Gebermedhin D., Medhora M., Roman R. J., Harder D. R. (1996). Molecular characterization of an arachidonic acid epoxygenase in rat brain astrocytes *Strkoe* 27:971-979.

Amruthesh S. C., Falck J. R., Ellis E. F. (1992).Brain synthesis and cerebrovascular action of epoxygenase metabolites of arachidonic acid. *J Neurochem* 58:503-510.

Amruthesh S. C., Boerschel M. F., McKinney J. S., Willoughby K. A., Ellis E. F. (1993).Metabolism of arachidonic acid to epoxyeicosatrienoic acids, hydroxyl-eicosatetraenoic acids, and prostaglandins in cultured rat hippocampal astrocytes.*J Neurochem* 61:150-159.

Anandatheerthavarada H. K., Shankar S. K., Ravindranath V.(1990). Rat brain cytochromes P450: catalytic, immunocytochemical properties and inducibility of multiple forms. *Brain Res.* 536:339-343.

Andreiuolo F., Junier M. P., Hol E. M., Miquel C., Chimelli L., Leonard N., Chneiweiss H., Daumas-Duport C., Varlet P. (2009). GFAP deltaimmunostaining improves visualization of normal and pathologic astrocytic heterogeneity. *Neuropathology* 29:31-39.

Arand M., Muller F., Mecky A., Hinz W., Urban P., Pompon D. (1999) Catalytic triad of microsomal epoxidehydrolase: replacement of glu404 with asp leads to a strongly increased turnover rate. *Biochem J* 337:37–43.

Bachoo R. M., Kim R. S., Ligon K. L., Maher E. A., Brennan C., Billings N., Chan S., Li C, Rowitch D. H., Wong W. H., Depinho R. A. (2004). Molecular diversity of astrocytes with implications for neurological disorders *ProcNatlAcadSci USA*101:8384-8389.

Beck D. W., Vinters H. V., Hart M. N., Cancilla P. A. (1984) Glial cells influence polarity of the blood-brain barrier. *J NeuropatholExpNeurol* 43:219-224.

Beetham J. K., Tian T., Hammock B. D. (1993) cDNA cloning and expression of a soluble epoxide hydrolase from humanliver. *Arch BiochemBiophys* 305:197–201.

Blechingberg J., Holm I. E., Nielsen K. B., Jensen T. H., Jorgensen A. L.., Neilsen A. L. (2007). Identification and characterization of GFAPkappa, a novel glial fibrillary acidic protein isoform.*Glia*55:497-507.

Brown A. M., Ransom B. R. (2007) Astrocyte glycogen and brain energy metabolism. *Glia* 55:1263-1271.

Burgener J., Falck J. R., Fritschy J. M., Arand M. (2009) Distribution of soluble and microsomal epoxide hydrolase in the mouse brain and its contribution to cerebral epoxyeicosatrienoic acid metabolism. *Neuroscience* 163(2):646-61.

Bush T. G., Savidge T. C., Freeman T. C., Cox H. J., Campbell E. A., Mucke L, Johnson MH, Sofroniew MV (1998). Fulminanntjejuno-ilritis following ablation of enteric glia in adult transgenic mice. *Cell* 93:189-201.

Capdevilla J., Chacos N., Werringloer J., Prough R., and Eastabrook R. (1982) Liver microsomal cytochrome P450 and oxidative metabolism of arachidonic acid. *Proc Natl.Acad Sci USA* 78:5362-5366.

Capdevilla J. H., Falk J. R. (2002). Biochemical and molecular properties of the cytochrome P450 arachidonic acid monooxygenases. *Prostaglandins Other lipid Mediat.* 68-69:325-344.

Charles A. C., Merrill J. E., Dirksen E. R., Sanderson M. J. (1991). Intercellular signaling in glial cells: calcium waves and oscillations in response to mechanical stimulation and glutamate. *Neuron* 6:983-992.

Chiamvimonvat N., Ho C., Tsai H., Hammock B. D. (2007) The soluble epoxide hydrolase as a pharmaceutical target for hypertension. *J Cardiovasc Pharmacol* 50:225-237.

Craft J. A., Baird S., Lamont M., Burchell B. (1990) Membrane topology of epoxide hydrolase.*BiochimBiophysActa* 1046:32–9.

Ellis E. F., Police R. .J, Yancey L., Mckinney J. S., Amruthesh S. C. (1990) Dilation of cerebral arterioles by cytochrome P-450 metabolites of arachidonic acid. *Am J Physiol* 259: H1171-H1177.

Eng L. F., Ghirnikar R. S., Lee Y. L. ( 2000) Glial fibrillary acidic protein: GFAP-thirty-one years (1969-2000). *Neurochem Res* 25:1439-1451.

Escortin C., Bonvento G. (2008) Targeted activation of astrocytes:a potential neuroprotective strategy. *MolNeurobiol* 38:231-241.

Fadda F., Rossetti Z. L. (1998) Chronic ethanol consumption: from neuroadaptation to neurodegeneration. *Prog.Neurobiol.* 56:385-431.

Faulkner J. R. , Hermann J. E., Woo M. J., Tansey K. E., Doan N. B., Sofroniew M. V.( 2004). Reactive astrocytes protect tissue and preserve function after spinal cord injury. *J Neurosci* 24:2143-2155.

Friedberg T., Lollmann B., Becker R., Holler R., Oesch F. (1994) The microsomal epoxide hydrolase has a singlemembrane signal anchor sequence which is dispensable for the catalytic activity of this protein. *Biochem J* 303(Pt 3):967–72.

Gegelashvili G., Civenni G., Racagni G., Danbolt N. C., Schousboe I., Schousboe A. (1996) Glutamate receptor agonists up-regulate glutamate transporter GLAST in astrocytes. *Neuroreport*20;8(1):261-5.

Ghersi-Egea J. F., Leninger-Muller B., Suleman G, Siest G., Minn A. (1994) Localization of drug-metabolizing enzymeactivities to blood–brain interfaces and circumventricular organs. *J Neurochem* 62:1089–96.

Goncalves C. A., Leite M. C., Nardin P. (2008) Biological and methodological featuresof the measurement of S100B, a putative marker of brain injury.*Clinical Biochem* 41:755-763.

Halassa M. M., Fellin T., Haydon P. G. (2007).The tripartite synapse:roles for gliotransmission in health disease. *Trends Mol Med* 13:54-63.

Hertz L., Peng L., Lai J. C. K. (1998) Functional studies in cultured astrocytes. *Methods* 16:293-310.

Howard L. A., MiKsys S., Hoffman E., Mash D., Tyndale R. F. (2003). Brain CYP2E1 is induced by nicotine and ethanol in rat and is highr in smokers and alcoholics. *Br J Pharmacol.* 138: 1376-1386.

Iadecola C., Nedergaard M. (2007) Glial regulation of the cerebral microvasculature. *Nat Neurosci* 10:1369-1376.

Iliff J. J., Alkayed N. J. (2009) Soluble epoxide hydrolase inhibition:targeting multiple mechanisms of ischemic brain injury with a single agent. *Future Neurol* 4:179-199.

Imig J. D., Hammock B. D. (2009) Soluble epoxide hydrolase as a therapeutic target for cardiovascular diseases. *Nat Rev Drug Discov* 8:794-805.

Inceoglu B., JinksS. L.,Ulu A., Hegedus C. M., Georgi K., Schmelzer K. R., Wagner K., Jones P. D., MorisseauC., HammockB. D. (2008) Soluble Epoxidehydrolase and epoxyeicosatrinenoic acids modulate two distinct analgesic pathways. *ProcNatlAcdSci USA*105:18901-18906.

Jackson M. R., Craft J. A., Burchell B. (1987) Nucleotide and deduced amino acid sequence of human liver microsomalepoxide hydrolase. *Nucleic Acids Res* 15:7188.

Kimelberg H. K., Nedergaard M. (2010) Functions of astrocytes and their potential as therapeutic targets. *Neurotherapeutics* 7:338-353.

Lacourciere G. M., Vakharia V. N., Tan C. P., Morris D. I., Edwards G. H., Moos M. (1993) Interaction of hepaticmicrosomal epoxide hydrolase derived from a recombinant baculovirus expression system with anazarene oxideand an aziridine substrate analogue. *Biochemistry* 32:2610–6.

Lieber C. S.(1999).Microsomal ethanol-oxidizing system (MEOS): the first 30 years (1968-1998) –review, Alcohol., *ClinExp Res* 23:991-1007.

Liu M., Alkayed N. J. (2005) Hypoxic preconditioning and tolerance via hypoxia inducible factor (HIF01 alpha-linked induction of P450C11 epoxygenase in astrocytes. *J Cereb Blood Flow Metab* 25:939-948.

McGiff J. C., Quilley J. (1999). 20-HETE and the kidney: resolution of old problems and new beginnings. *Am J Physiol* 277:R607-623.

Meyer R. P., Gehlhaus M., Knoth R., Volk B. (2007). Expression and function of cytochrome p450 in brain drug metabolism. *Curr Drug Metab.* 8(4):297-306.

Michealis U. R., Fisslthaler B., Barosa-Sicard E., Falck J. R., Fleming I., Busse R. (2005) Cytochrome P450 epoxygenases 2C8 and 2C9 are implicated in hypoxia-induced endothelial cell migration and angiogensis. *J cell Sci* 118:5489-5498.

Miksys S., Rao Y., Hoffman E., Mash D. C., Tyndole R. F. (2002).Regional and cellular expression of CYP2D6 inhuman brain: higher levels in alcoholics. *J. Neurochem.* 82:1376-1387.

Miksys S., Lerman C., Shields P. G., Mash D. C., Tyndole R. F.(2003). Smoking alcoholism and genetic polymorphisms alter CYPB6 levels in human brain. *Neuropharmacology* 45:122-132.

Miksys S., Tyndole R. F. 2004 The unique regulation of brain cytochromeP450 2 (CYP2) family enzymes by drugs and genetics. *Drug Metabol Rev.* 36:313-333.

Morisseau C., Hammock B. D. (2005) Epoxide hydrolases: mechanisms, inhibitor designs, and biological roles. *Annu Rev Pharmacol Toxicol*45:311-333.

Nedergaard M., Ransom B., Goldman S. A. (2003) New roles for aastrocytes: redefining the functional architecture of the brain. *Trends Neurosci* 32:189-198.

Newman J. W., Morisseau C., Harris T. R., Hammock B. D. (2003) The soluble epoxide hydrolase encoded by EPXH2 is abifunctional enzyme with novel lipid phosphate phosphatase activity. *ProcNatlAcadSci USA* 100:1558–63.

Newman J. W., Morisseau C., Harris T. R., Hammock B. D. (2005) Epoxide hydrolases:their roles and interactions with lipidmetabolism. *Prog Lipid Res* 44:1-51.

Norenberg M. D. (1979) Distribution of glutamine synthetase in the rat central nervous system. *J Histochem Cytochem* 27:756-762.

Ohe T., Hirobe M., MashinoT. (2000). Novel metabolic pathway of estrone and 17beta-estradiol catalyzed by cytochrome-P450. *Drug Metabol Dispos* 28:110-112.

Pekny M., Pekna M. (2004) astrocyte intermediate filaments in CNS pathologies and regeneration. *J Pathol* 204:428-437.

Peters A., Palay S. L., Webster H. D. (1991) The fine structures of the nervous system, Third edn. Oxford University Press, New York.

Perea G., Navarrette M., Araque A. (2009)Tripartitesynapses:astrocytes process and control synaptic information. *Trends Neurosci* 32:t421-t431.

Revermann M., Barbosa-Sicard E., Dony E., Schermuly R. T., Morisseau C., Geisslinger G., Fleming I., Hammock B. D., Brandes R. P. (2009) Inhibiton of the soluble epoxide hydrolase attenuates monocrotaline-induced pulmonary hypertension in rats. *J Hypertens* 27:322-331.

Roman R. J. (2002). P-450 metabolites of arachidonic acid in the control of cardiovascular function. Physiol Rev 82:131-185.

Rosenbrock H., Hagemeyer C. E., Singec I., Knoth R., Volk B. (2001). Expression and localization of the CYP2B subfamily predominantly in neurons of rat brain. *J. Neurochem.*76:332-340

Ruhl A. (2005) Glial cells in the gut. *Neurogastroenterol Motil* 17:777-790.

Sattler R., Rothstein J. D. (2006) Regulation and dysregulation of glutamate transporters. *HandbExpPharmacol* 175:277-303.

Schladt L., Wörner W., Setiabudi F., Oesch F. (1986) Distribution and inducibility of cytosolic epoxide hydrolase in male Sprague-Dawley rats. BiochemPharmacol35 (19):3309-16.

Schmelzer K. R., Kubala L., Newman J. W., Kim I. H., Eiserich J. P., Hammock B. D. (2005) Soluble epoxide hydrolase is atherapeutic target for acute inflammation. *Proc Natl Acad Sci USA* 102:9772-9777.

Seifert G., Schilling K., Steinhauser C. (2006) Astrocytes dysfunction in neurological disorders: a molecular perspective. *Nat Rev Neurosci* 7:194-206.

Shigetomi E., Bowser D. N., Sofroniew M. V., Khakh B. S. (2003) Two forms of astrocytye calcium excitability have distinct effects on NMDA receptor-mediated slow inwardcurrents in pyramidal neurons. *J Neurosci* 28:6659-6663.

Shivachar A. C., Willoughby K. A., Ellis E. F. (1995) Effect of protein kinase C modulators on 14,15-EET incorporation into astroglial phospholipids. *J Neurochem* 65:338-346.

Smith K. R., Pinkerton K. E., Watanabe T., Pederson T. L., Ma S. J., Hammock B. D. (2005) Attenuationof Tobacco smoke-induced lung inflammation by treatmentwith a soluble epoxide hydrolase inhibitor. *ProcNatlAcadSci* USA 102:2186-2191.

Sofroniew M. V., Vinters H. V. (2010) Astrocytes: biology and pathology. *ActaNeuropathol* 119:7-35.

Somjen G. G. (1988) Nervenkitt: notes on the history of the concept of microglia. *Glia* 1:2-9.

Takano T., Oberheim N., Cotrina M. L., Nedergaard M. (2009) Astrocytes and Ischemic injury. *Stroke*40:S8-12.

Taura Ki K., Yamada H., Naito E., Ariyoshi N., Mori Ma M. A., Oguri K. (2002). Activation of microsomal epoxidehydrolase by interaction with cytochromes P450: kinetic analysis of the association and substrate-specificactivation of epoxide hydrolase function. *Arch Biochem Biophys*402:275–80.

Teissier E., Fennrich S., Strazielle N., Daval J. L., Ray D., Schlosshauer B. (1998) Drug metabolism in invitro organotypic and cellular models of mammalian central nervous system: activities of membraneboundepoxide hydrolase and NADPH-cytochrome P-450 (c) reductase. *Neurotoxicology* 19:347–55.

Thrane A. S., Rappold P. M., Fujita T., Torres A., Bekar L. K., Takano T., Peng W., Wang F., Thrane V. R., Enger R., Haj-yaseen N. N., Skare O., Holen T., Klungland A., Otterson O. P., Nedergaard M., Nagelhus E. A. (2011). Criticalroleofaquaporin-4 inastrocyticCa$^{++}$ signaling events elicited by cerebraledema. *ProcNatlAcadSci USA* 108:846-851.

Volk B., Meyer R. P., Lintig F. V., Ibach B., Knoth R. (1995) Localization and Characterization of cytochrome 450 in the brain. In vivo and in vitro investigations on phenytoin- and Phenobarbital-inducible forms. *Toxicol.Lett.* 82/83:655-622.

Voltera A., Meldolesi J. (2005) Astrocytes from brain glue to communication elements:the revolution continues. *Nat Rev Neurosci* 6:626-640.

Warner M., Gustafsson J. A. (1994) Effect of ethanol on cytochrome P450 in the rat brain. *ProcNatlAcadSci USA*. 9:1019-1023.

Yamaura K., Gebermedhin D., Zhang C., Narayanan , Hoefert K., Jacobs E. R., Koehler R. C., Harder D. R. (2006) Contribution of epoxyeicosatrienoic acids to the hypoxia-induced activation of Ca$^{++}$ activated K$^{+}$ channel current in cultured rat hippocampal astrocytes. *Neuroscience* 143:703-716.

Yang B., Graham L., Dikalov S., Mason R. P., Falck J. R., Lia J. K., Zeldin D. C. (2001) Overexpression of cytochrome P450 CYP2J2 protects against hypoxia-reoxygenation injury in cultured bovine aortic endothelial cells. *MolPharmacol* 60:310-320.

Zhang W., Koerner I. P., Noppens R., Grafe M., Tsai H. J., Morisseau C., Luria A., Hammock B. D., Falck J. R., Alkayed N. J. (2007) Solubleepoxide hydrolase: a novel therapeutic target in stroke. *J Cereb Blood Flow Metab* 27:1931–1940.

Zhang W.,OtsukaT., Sugo N., Ardeshri A., Alhadid Y. K., Iliff J. J., DeBarber A. E., Koop D. R., Alkayed N. J. (2008) Soluble epoxide hydrolase gene deletion isprotective against experimental cerebral ischemia. *Stroke* 39:2073-2078.

Zhanger U. M., Raimundo S., Eichelbaum M. (2004) Cytochrome P450 2D6: overview and update on pharmacology genetics, biochemistry. *Naunyn-Schmiederg's Arch Pharmacol.* 369:23-37.

In: Astrocytes
Editor: Oscar González-Pérez

ISBN: 978-1-62081-558-8
© 2012 Nova Science Publishers, Inc.

*Chapter II*

# Astrocytic Potassium Channels in Central Nervous System Disorders

*Miroslava Anderova* and Helena Pivonkova*
Department of Cellular Neurophysiology, Institute of Experimental Medicine,
Academy of Sciences of the Czech Republic, Videnska, Prague, Czech Republic

## Abstract

Astrocytes are particularly complex cells responding to a large number of stimuli, such as extra/intracellular ion concentration shifts, pH shifts or increased neurotransmitter and hormone levels. Under physiological conditions, one of their key functions is to maintain ionic homeostasis in the brain during neuronal activity by a process called potassium spatial buffering. Several mechanisms are believed to underlie the maintenance of $K^+$ homeostasis, among which astrocytic $K^+$ conductances play an important role. Potassium spatial buffering is based on the expression of weakly inwardly rectifying $K^+$ (Kir) channels, predominantly Kir4.1, which enable the high $K^+$ permeability of the plasma membrane and establish a strongly negative resting membrane potential in astrocytes. Additionally, two-pore domain $K^+$ channels, namely TREK1, 2 and TWIK1, which are also highly expressed in astrocytes, might play a significant role in $K^+$ spatial buffering due to their constitutive open state allowing "passive" $K^+$ ion fluxes. Recent data indicate that the expression and functioning of astrocytic $K^+$ channels are seriously affected under many acute and chronic pathological conditions. In particular, a $K^+$ inward current decreases together with reduced Kir4.1 channel expression or Kir4.1 channel mislocation have been shown in both the retina and the brain after an insult. These changes are accompanied by astrocytic depolarization, ultimately leading to impaired $K^+$ buffering, and also to a decreased ability of astrocytes to clear excess extracellular glutamate, both of which contribute to ongoing damage of the nervous tissue. In this review, we focus on summarizing current knowledge about the expression and functioning of $K^+$ channels in astrocytes during the acute and chronic stages of CNS disorders, such as ischemia or epilepsy. The role of other proteins that might functionally interact with $K^+$ channels and influence $K^+$ buffering during CNS disorders, namely aquaporins and connexins, will also be discussed.

---

*E-Mail: anderova@biomed.cas.cz.

## Introduction

Astrocytes represent a far more interesting glial cell type then one would have imagined only several decades ago. They make up about 30% of the cellular population in the rodent brain, and they even outnumber neurons in phylogenetically higher species, such as in humans (Nedergaard et al., 2003). Such high astrocyte density implies that they constitute a functionally essential part of the nervous tissue, especially in more elaborated brains. Indeed, during the last decades, many unexpected astrocytic functions have been described; for example, modulation of synaptic transmission (Haydon, 2001), an intrinsic mean of communication by $Ca^{2+}$ waves (Cornell-Bell and Finkbeiner, 1991), regulation of blood flow through the brain microvessels (Gordon et al., 2007) and even cells with astrocytic properties acting as stem cells in the neurogenic regions of the adult brain (Doetsch et al., 1999; Seri et al., 2004; Menn et al., 2006; Wang and Bordey, 2008). Regardless of all of these astrocytic functions, proper neuronal activity essentially depends on the ability of astrocytes to maintain ionic and neurotransmitter homeostasis in the nervous tissue, which is primarily accomplished by the clearance of extracellular $K^+$ and glutamate extruded from neurons into the extracellular space (ECS) during their physiological activity (Kofuji and Newman, 2004). To fulfill their role in maintaining $K^+$ homeostasis in the brain, astrocytes express several types of $K^+$ ion channels, which are endowed with suitable properties for $K^+$ clearance from the ECS.

Acute pathological states of the nervous tissue, such as ischemia, traumatic brain injury or seizures, are characterized by impaired ionic homeostasis accompanied by the accumulation of $K^+$ ions and glutamate in the ECS (Muller and Somjen, 2000; Homola et al., 2006). Based on morphological studies, astrocytes give the impression that they are the last cell type to respond to injury after neurons or oligodendrocytes, which die soon after insult, but astrocytes mostly survive and change into a stage called reactive glia (Fawcett and Asher, 1999). However, the functional response of astrocytes to the ionic imbalance must be prompt and is characterized by $K^+$ uptake followed by cell swelling (Leis et al., 2005). The main role in this process is played by $K^+$ ion channels allowing $K^+$ influx into astrocytes. Depending on the extent, duration and type of the injury, astrocytes might, using this mechanism, protect the affected nervous tissue from the consequences of the ionic disbalance (Swanson et al., 2004). Interestingly, during late stages of central nervous system (CNS) injuries, the mechanism of $K^+$ clearance by astrocytes seems to be impaired because of changes in the expression and/or functioning of the astrocytic $K^+$ ion channels.

In our chapter, we focus on the role of astrocytic $K^+$ channels during the pathogenesis of some common CNS disorders. We try to address the question whether astrocytes might be able to fulfill their homeostatic functions after CNS injury in terms of the $K^+$ spatial buffering mechanism and $K^+$ channel activity. Since controversy exists about the heterogeneity of astrocytes, we specifically focus on mature "passive" astrocytes in the adult brain that display high $K^+$ permeability and high Kir4.1 channel expression, form large syncytium and are thus primarily responsible for $K^+$ spatial buffering. This astrocytic population seems to be relatively homogeneous (Mishima and Hirase, 2010).

## Physiological Functions of $K^+$ Ion Channels in Astrocytes

### The Types of $K^+$ Ion Channels Expressed in Astrocytes

Mature astrocytes express predominantly two types of $K^+$ ion channels – inwardly rectifying $K^+$ (Kir) channels and two-pore domain $K^+$ ($K_{2P}$) channels (Seifert et al., 2009; Zhou et al., 2009). Kir channels are widely expressed in many cell types and play an important role in diverse physiological functions in the brain, retina, ears, heart, kidney and endocrine cells. The 15 known members of the Kir channel family are divided based on their electrophysiological and molecular characteristics into 7 subfamilies (Kir1-7) (Kubo et al., 2005; Hibino et al., 2010). The primary function of Kir channels is maintaining the cell resting membrane potential (RMP) hyperpolarized close to the equilibrium potential for $K^+$ ($E_K$). In excitable cells, such as cardiomyocytes or neurons, Kir channels thus contribute to the modulation of cell excitability and action potential repolarization. Kir channels form tetrameric structures, which can be co-assembled by heteromeric or homomeric Kir subunits. Each subunit has two transmembrane segments called M1 and M2, a pore loop (P), and amino (N)- and carboxy (C)-terminal cytoplasmic domains (for review see Bichet et al., 2003). The selectivity filter of the Kir channel, defined as the narrowest part of the conduction pathway, primarily discriminates between $K^+$ and $Na^+$ ions. The determining feature of Kir channels is their ability to conduct $K^+$ better in the inward than in the outward direction. The inward rectification of Kir channels is caused by blocking the channel by intracellular $Mg^{2+}$ and/or polyamines (e.g., putrescine, spermine, spermidine) at potentials positive to the cell RMP, thus impeding the outward flow of $K^+$ ions. Another characteristic feature of inward rectification is its strong voltage dependence. Based on the degree of rectification correlating with the binding affinity of the channel for blocking cations, we can distinguish weak (Kir1, Kir4, Kir6) and strong (Kir2, Kir3) rectifiers. The activity of Kir channels might be modulated by several cytoplasmic factors, namely phosphatidylinositol-4,5-bisphosphate (PtdIns (4,5)P2), arachidonic acid (AA), $Na^+$ and $Mg^{2+}$ ions, pH, G proteins, adenosine-5'-triphosphate (ATP), phosphorylation or oxidation/reduction. PtdIns(4, 5)P2 enhances the currents through Kir channels; on the other hand, its depletion during patch-clamp measurements, similarly to ATP, causes the channel to rundown (Bichet et al., 2003).

Astrocytes have been shown to express a wide range of Kir channels (Butt and Kalsi, 2006), although mature astrocytes in the adult CNS show a predominant and specific expression of the Kir4.1 isoform (Poopalasundaram et al., 2000; Seifert et al., 2009), which is believed to represent the prerequisite for the high $K^+$ conductance in astrocytes, setting their RMP close to $E_K$ and allowing the $K^+$ buffering mechanism to function. The currents through Kir channels are modulated by the extracellular $K^+$ concentration ($[K^+]_e$), which permits greater $K^+$ uptake when $[K^+]_e$ is raised. Kir4.1 forms functional heteromeric channels with Kir2.1 and Kir5.1 subunits in astrocytes (Hibino et al., 2004), which display specific features such as higher sensitivity to changes in intracellular pH (Cui et al., 2001) and stronger rectification compared to homomeric Kir4.1 channels.

$K_{2P}$ channels are the last family of $K^+$ channels, discovered only in the 1990s. As their name indicates, these channels are characterized by a specific subunit topology, i.e., two P loops and four transmembrane segments. Biophysical experiments on $K_{2P}$ channels revealed that they are $K^+$ selective with voltage-independent conductance that obeys Goldman-Hodgkin-Katz (open) rectification. Thus, these channels have been suggested to be responsible for the background $K^+$ conductance in many cell types. When the $K^+$

concentration is symmetrical across the membrane, $K_{2P}$ channels conduct $K^+$ currents in a linear manner, while under physiological $K^+$ concentrations, they pass greater outward than inward currents. These properties give $K_{2P}$ channels significant physiological functions – they maintain the RMP of many cell types and regulate the activity of neurons and other excitable cells (Goldstein et al., 2001). Many members of the $K_{2P}$ channel family display polymodal characteristics, i.e., they are activated and/or modulated by different stimuli, for example, volatile anesthetics, AA, temperature, pH or mechanical stress, which might be important during many pathological processes (Honore, 2007).

Since astrocytes *in situ* display large passive, i.e., voltage-independent $K^+$ currents, it has been speculated that these currents might be based on the constitutive opening of $K_{2P}$ channels. Indeed, the expression of this type of $K^+$ channel has been shown recently in both cultured astrocytes as well as in astrocytes *in situ*. In cultured cortical astrocytes, Ferroni et al. (2003) have shown the expression of an open rectifier $K^+$ channel activated by AA, presumably of the TREK family. Similar results were published by Gnatenco et al. (2002) using single-channel patch-clamp recording. These preliminary results have been recently verified by two groups who showed the expression of $K_{2P}$ channels in hippocampal astrocytes *in situ*. These researchers demonstrated that passive $K^+$ conductance in astrocytes *in situ* is mediated by the combined expression of Kir4.1 channels together with the $K_{2P}$ channels TWIK1 and TREK1 (Seifert et al., 2009; Zhou et al., 2009).

### Spatial $K^+$ Buffering

Physiological neuronal activity results in the extrusion of $K^+$ ions into the ECS, leading to changes in the electrochemical gradients across their membranes and their subsequent depolarization. $[K^+]_e$ thus modulates the excitability of neurons, and its increase might lead to neuronal hyperactivity and synchronous discharges followed by epileptic seizures (Trachtenberg and Pollen, 1970). Under physiological conditions or near physiological stimulation, $[K^+]_e$ increases from 3mM by ~0.5mM (Somjen, 2002). Intensive stimulation or seizures leads to a $[K^+]_e$ rise up to a ceiling level of ~10-12mM (Heinemann and Lux, 1977), while during ischemia or spreading depression $[K^+]_e$ might elevate even up to 80mM (Somjen GG, 2002). The first well characterized astrocytic function is their maintenance of ionic homeostasis in the nervous tissue. Kuffler et al. (1966) and Orkand et al. (1966) demonstrated the high $K^+$ permeability of the glial cell membrane and active neuronal-glial interactions by showing that stimulation of the amphibian optic nerve triggered the depolarization of the adjacent glia. Since astrocytes possess large $K^+$ conductance and thus their membrane potential lies close to $E_K$, astrocytes sense slight changes in $[K^+]_e$ produced by firing neurons. Based on these findings, Orkand (1986) proposed a hypothesis of $K^+$ spatial buffering, which was later elaborated in more detail by Kofuji and Newman (2004). Astrocytes, being perfect $K^+$ concentration sensors, follow changes in $[K^+]_e$, which increases during a higher rate of neuronal firing, by subtle changes in their membrane potential. Potassium ions are taken up into astrocytes at sites of high neuronal activity and are redistributed through the astrocyte syncytium. $K^+$ ions are then extruded at sites of relative low $K^+$ concentration. Other mechanisms contributing to $K^+$ ion homeostasis are net $K^+$ and $Cl^-$ uptake by specific ion channels and/or transporters and $K^+$ uptake via $Na^+K^+ATPase$ (Walz, 2000).

The $K^+$ spatial buffering mechanism is based on the polarized expression of specific ion channels on the astrocytic membrane. The subcellular expression of the weak inwardly rectifying $K^+$ channel, Kir4.1, has a distinct spatial pattern – Kir4.1 is expressed on astrocytic endfeet surrounding synapses and blood vessels. Since Kir4.1 is a weakly rectifying channel and may thus allow $K^+$ fluxes in both directions, it is perfectly suited for functioning in the $K^+$ buffering mechanism. On the other hand, Kir2.1 is expressed only on astrocyte membranes surrounding neuronal synapses. It is a strongly rectifying channel, and thus it allows only an inward flow of $K^+$ ions, which are further redistributed through the astrocytic syncytium (Newman, 1986). A similar mechanism as $K^+$ spatial buffering, $K^+$ siphoning, has been well described in retinal Muller cells. Potassium siphoning occurs within one Muller cell. Potassium is taken up by strongly rectifying Kir2.1 channels at processes close to neuronal synapses, then redistributed throughout the Muller cell and extruded by weakly rectifying Kir4.1 channels at processes near the vitreous body and retinal blood vessels (Kofuji et al., 2002). The involvement of other Kir or $K_{2P}$ channels in $K^+$ spatial buffering is still a matter of debate. Pasler et al. (2007) have shown that quinine/quinidine-sensitive $K_{2P}$ channels might possibly contribute to glial $K^+$ buffering.

## *The Effect of Pharmacological and Genetic Inactivation of $K^+$ Channels on Astrocyte Functions*

For many years it has been speculated that glial Kir channel currents are well suited for the removal of extracellular $K^+$ excess following neuronal activity (Newman et al., 1984; Newman, 1986; Ransom and Sontheimer, 1995). However, pharmacological studies using $Ba^{2+}$ and $Cs^+$ as Kir channel blockers have brought many controversial results about the role of Kir channels in $K^+$ spatial buffering. In the presence of 0.5 mM $Ba^{2+}$, the usual depolarizing response of glial cells in the guinea pig olfactory cortex to a rise in extracellular $K^+$ activity reversed into a membrane hyperpolarization. Furthermore, $Ba^{2+}$ strongly reduced the stimulus-related rise of intra-glial $K^+$ accumulation (Ballanyi et al., 1987). D'Ambrosio and colleagues showed that glial Kir channels are involved in the regulation of baseline levels of $K^+$ and in decreasing the amplitude of the post-activity $[K^+]_e$ undershoot, but they do not affect the rate of $K^+$ clearance during neuronal firing (D'Ambrosio et al., 2002). On the other hand, barium did not significantly affect resting $[K^+]_e$ or the $[K^+]_e$ rises detected by a $K^+$-sensitive electrode after short-stimulus trains (Meeks and Mennerick, 2007). These discrepancies probably result from the fact that neither $Ba^{2+}$ nor $Cs^+$ act as specific blockers of Kir channels. Barium at higher concentrations also blocks $K_{2P}$ channels and $Cs^+$ might cross $K_{2P}$ channels opened at rest in glia. These methodological shortcomings have been overcome by creating transgenic mice lacking genes for specific ion channels, in which the significance of a defined channel in $K^+$ spatial buffering can be investigated.

The first Kir4.1 knockout mouse was generated by Paolo Kofuji and colleagues, and the role of these channels in the regulation of extracellular $K^+$ was shown in the retina (Kofuji et al., 2000). It seems that Kir4.1 and astrocytes play a very specific role in the process of $K^+$ removal after neuronal activity. Neusch et al. (2006) showed that a lack of Kir4.1 channel subunits in astrocytes in the ventral respiratory group of the brain stem did not influence the basic neuronal activity, although the baseline of $[K^+]_e$ in Kir4.1$^{-/-}$ mice was higher and the decay of a stimulus-induced increase of $[K^+]_e$ was slower and exhibited an undershoot. This result is in line with previous results shown by D'Ambrosio et al. (2002), who demonstrated that the stimulus-induced increase in $[K^+]_e$ is cleared by neuronal and glial $Na^+K^+ATPase$ together with glial Kir channels. The observed undershoot is due to the prolonged activity of the $Na^+K^+ATPase$, and under normal conditions, this decrease in $[K^+]_e$ is replenished by the release of $K^+$ through Kir channels. Conditional knock-out of the Kir4.1 gene in adult astrocytes leads to their depolarization, the inhibition of $K^+$ and glutamate uptake and subsequent $K^+$ accumulation in the extracellular space (Djukic et al., 2007; Kucheryavykh et al., 2007). Recently, the pivotal role of Kir4.1 channels for efficient $K^+$ spatial buffering has been confirmed by *in vivo* data obtained in transgenic animals lacking astrocytic Kir 4.1 expression (Chever et al., 2010). The impact of knocking out other astrocytic channels, for instance, Kir2.1, Kir2.2, Kir2.3, Kir5.1 or $K_{2P}$ channels, on $K^+$ buffering has not yet been investigated.

## *Functional Interactions with Other Channels Involved in $K^+$ Buffering*

Recently, the question of functional cooperation between different types of ion channels has been put forward. In astrocytes, co-localization and functional interaction are known between Kir4.1 channels and aquaporin-4 (AQP4) water channels. Aquaporins, in general, allow water movement through hydrophobic membranes (Verkman, 2005). Subcellular AQP4 channel distribution in astrocytes mimics that of Kir4.1 channels, i.e., they are both enriched at the endfeet contacting brain microvessels and the subarachnoidal space (Nagelhus et al., 1999; Nagelhus et al., 2004). It has been shown that AQP4 mislocation in α-syntrophin knockout mice leads to impaired $K^+$ clearance from the ECS (Amiry-Moghaddam et al., 2003), indicating that ion movement through Kir channels is facilitated by water movement through aquaporins.

Since the redistribution of $K^+$ ions during $K^+$ spatial buffering from sites of its high to sites of its low concentration is ultimately dependent on a functional astroglial syncytium (Kofuji and Newman, 2004), it is apparent that the impairment of astrocytic connections by gap junctions might influence $K^+$ clearance from the ECS under physiological as well as pathological conditions. It has been shown that mice lacking Cx43 in their astrocytes, with significantly reduced intercellular dye coupling, show a deficient redistribution of $K^+$ ions leading to an increased velocity of wave propagation during spreading depression (Theis et al., 2003). Similar results were published later showing that astrocytic gap junctions accelerate $K^+$ clearance, limit $K^+$ accumulation during synchronized neuronal firing, and aid in radial $K^+$ relocation in the hippocampus.

Furthermore, brain slices of mice with coupling-deficient astrocytes displayed a reduced threshold for the generation of epileptiform events, although gap junction-dependent processes only partially account for $K^+$ buffering in the hippocampus (Wallraff et al., 2006).

Astrocytes are the cell type primarily responsible for glutamate clearance from the ECS after neuronal activity. An increase in the extracellular glutamate concentration during acute pathological states in the CNS is suggested to play a role in seizure generation. Astrocytes express two types of glutamate transporters – EAAT1 (GLAST) and EAAT2 (GLT1) – which use the transmembrane electrochemical gradients of $Na^+$ and $K^+$ ions to transport glutamate against its electrochemical gradient into the cells.

Glutamate clearance by astrocytes is thus directly dependent on maintaining physiological $K^+$ concentrations in the nervous tissue and the hyperpolarized RMP in astrocytes. Indeed, several studies have shown that glutamate uptake is impaired after Kir4.1 channel knock-down and subsequent astrocyte depolarization (Djukic et al., 2007; Kucheryavykh et al., 2007).

## Alterations in K⁺ Channel Expression and Function in CNS Disorders

For decades, a large number of studies has focused on the role of neurons in CNS disorders; however, it is becoming increasingly evident that glial cells, which play an irreplaceable role in brain homeostasis and synaptic plasticity, might profoundly influence pathophysiological processes as well. Since astrocytic K⁺ channels represent a prerequisite for the maintenance of K⁺ homeostasis, a large number of studies has focused on identifying changes in the expression of specific Kir channel subunits and their functioning in astroglial cells in response to pathological states of the CNS, such as neurodegenerative diseases, gliomas, epilepsy, trauma, ischemia or hepatic encephalopathy. Recently, attention has also turned to $K_{2P}$ channels, in addition to Kir channels, as these have been shown to contribute to the background leak K⁺ currents in astrocytes and to participate in maintaining K⁺ homeostasis. The astroglial reaction to CNS diseases/injuries appears to be uniform with respect to reactive astrocyte morphology, although the findings obtained in different models of CNS injury imply that alterations in the membrane properties of reactive astrocytes can differ due to the nature and the extent of CNS injury or neurodegenerative disease progression.

### *Neurodegenerative Diseases*

One of the most studied neurodegenerative diseases in terms of astrocytic K⁺ channels is Alzheimer's disease (AD). This progressive neurodegenerative disorder is characterized by extracellular amyloid deposits, intracellular neurofibrillary tangles and neuronal loss as well as by changes in astrocyte morphology (Olabarria et al., 2010) and astrocyte membrane properties (Wilcock et al., 2009). In transgenic mouse models of both moderate and severe vascular amyloid deposition with disease progression to tau pathology and neuronal loss, Wilcock and colleagues showed that the endfeet of perivascular astrocytes lack glial fibrilary acidic protein (GFAP) and, moreover, that Kir4.1 and calcium-sensitive large-conductance K⁺ (BK) channels are lost in the endfeet region together with water channels, namely AQP4. In addition, they demonstrated that the anchoring protein dystrophin 1 is also reduced in astrocytic endfeet in conjunction with AD progression. A similar pattern of Kir4.1, AQP4 and dystrophin 1 reduction was observed in autopsied brain tissue from AD patients that displayed moderate or severe vascular amyloid deposits (Wilcock et al., 2009). The same authors found an increase in mRNA and protein expression of the TASK2 channel, which is a $K_{2P}$ channel sensitive to changes in extracellular pH and is found in astrocytes (Rusznak et al., 2004). Taken together, the loss of Kir4.1 and AQP4 indicates impaired K⁺ buffering and water transport during AD progression. Electrophysiological studies describing the impact of AD progression on astrocytic K⁺ channels are rare. Increased activation of both K⁺ and Cl⁻ channels by small concentrations of beta-amyloid protein was described in cultured neonatal astrocytes, indicating the disturbance of ionic homeostasis in astrocytes before any profound visible peptide accumulation in the brain (Jalonen et al., 1997). Recently, increased astrocyte coupling in the neocortex of aged (20 to 27 months) amyloid-beta protein precursor overexpressing mice was described together with the increased expression of functional glutamate transporters and AMPA/kainate-type glutamate receptors (Peters et al., 2009). Similarly, in a model of amyotrophic lateral sclerosis, a progressive loss of the glial K⁺ channel Kir4.1 in the ventral horn of the spinal cord was demonstrated by immunohistochemistry in transgenic mice expressing the superoxide dismutase G93A mutation SOD1 (G93A) (Kaiser et al., 2006). Immunoblotting of spinal cord extracts showed a loss of Kir4.1 channels from pre-symptomatic stages onwards, thus excluding astrogliosis as a primary cause of Kir4.1 down-regulation. Nevertheless, the membrane properties of astrocytes have rarely been investigated in the aged brain, and thus the role of astrocytes not only in AD, but also in other neurodegenerative disorders such as Parkinson's disease, Huntington's disease or amyotrophic lateral sclerosis, is poorly understood and needs to be elucidated.

*Gliomas*

In general, ion channels can also play an important role in cancer development and tumor outgrowth. In glial-derived tumors, certain $K^+$ channels, namely $Ca^{2+}$-activated $K^+$ channels, have received most of the interest (Kunzelmann, 2005). Nevertheless, the attention of researchers has also turned to glial Kir channels, because their increasing expression in glia was shown to correlate with a loss of cell proliferation and enhanced differentiation during development, suggesting their involvement in glial growth control. Western blot and reverse transcription polymerase chain reaction (PCR) analyses revealed the high expression of several Kir channel genes, including Kir2.1, 2.3, 3.1 and also 4.1, at the transcript and protein levels in glioma cells (Olsen and Sontheimer, 2004). In contrast to wild-type spinal cord astrocytes, in which Kir4.1 channels are expressed throughout the plasma membrane, in astrocytoma cells they are absent from the plasma membrane, but highly expressed in the nucleus (Olsen and Sontheimer, 2008). The first detailed analysis of the expression pattern of Kir4.1 in various human brain tumors was performed by Warth et al. (2005). They found an early mislocalization of Kir4.1 channel protein in various low- and high-grade human brain astrocytomas, which might lead to compromised $K^+$ transport in astroglial cells. Despite the fact that dystrophin expression was always restricted to the astrocytic endfeet in both low- and high-grade astrocytomas, AQP4 was redistributed only in high-grade astrocytomas, which implies that the clustering mechanisms of Kir4.1 and AQP4 are different. On the other hand, employing PCR, Western blot and immunohistochemistry Tan et al. (2008) investigated Kir4.1 mRNA and Kir4.1 protein expression in eighty cases of human astrocytic tumors. Interestingly, their data revealed that the expression of Kir4.1 mRNA and protein, as well as the Kir4.1 immunoreactivity increase markedly with increasing pathologic grade. Based on this finding, they proposed to use Kir4.1 as a new biomarker for astrocytic tumors.

Patch-clamp recordings revealed that there are no Kir currents in gliomas, while $Ca^{2+}$-activated $K^+$ channels have been detected (Ransom and Sontheimer, 2001). In low-grade pilocytic astrocytomas obtained from biopsies of 4-month- to 14-year-old pediatric patients, Bordey and Sontheimer (1998a) showed that astrocytoma cells almost exclusively display delayed rectifying $K^+$ currents and transient, tetrodotoxin-sensitive sodium currents; however, they lack transient "A"-type $K^+$ currents and Kir currents. On the other hand, $Ba^{2+}$-sensitive inwardly rectifying Kir channels were detected in the human malignant astrocytoma cell line U87-MG (Ducret et al., 2003). Of note, the transient or stable transfection of Kir4.1 channels in human glioma cells led to their functional expression, resulting in the arrest of cell growth, while blocking the inwardly rectifying current with $Ba^{2+}$ or depolarizing the glioma membrane by 20 mM $K^+$ resulted in the onset of proliferation (Olsen and Sontheimer, 2008). As Kir4.1 channels are expressed by differentiated, non-proliferating astrocytes, the idea of enhancing their expression in astrocytoma cells and their proper targeting to the cell

## Epilepsy

Since the astrocytic buffering of extracellular $K^+$ plays an important role in the regulation of neuronal excitability, an uncontrolled increase in $[K^+]_e$ leads to neuronal depolarization and hyperexcitability as well as anomalous synaptic transmission, and it ultimately results in seizure activity (Rothstein et al., 1996; Janigro et al., 1997; Tanaka et al., 1997; D'Ambrosio et al., 1998). As astroglial Kir channels have been proposed to play an important role in the maintenance of $K^+$ homeostasis, their properties have been studied in experimental and human epilepsy by several groups. Generally, their results have shown that the astrocytes surrounding seizure foci differ in their morphological and physiological properties when compared to astrocytes in healthy tissue, and that glial $K^+$ buffering might be impaired at the seizure foci due to the loss of Kir channel activity. Using the patch-clamp technique, the down-regulation of astrocytic Kir channels was first demonstrated by Bordey and Sontheimer (1998b) in acute slices of biopsies from patients undergoing surgery for intractable mesio-temporal lobe epilepsy and also in acute hippocampal slices from surgical specimens of patients suffering from pharmaco-resistant temporal lobe epilepsy (Hinterkeuser et al., 2000; Schroder et al., 2000). Similarly, the acute impairment of astroglial Kir channels and $K^+$ buffering was described after a fluid percussion injury, a model simulating human contusive closed head injury and post-traumatic epilepsy (D'Ambrosio et al., 1999). Recently, Stewart et al. (2010) showed a decrease in Kir4.1 channel expression in the rat neocortex after a fluid percussion injury connected with the chronic impairment of Kir currents in astrocytes in the epileptic focus. Accordingly, reduced Kir4.1 channel activity in astrocytes associated with deficits in $K^+$ and glutamate buffering was also found in the hippocampus of seizure-susceptible mice (Inyushin et al., 2010). Besides all of these changes in Kir4.1 expression/function, the increased expression of the Kir2.1 channel subunit was detected in hippocampal astrocytes 3-5 days after kainic acid-induced seizure (Kang et al., 2008). These immunohistochemical findings imply that astrocytic Kir2.1 channels might be also involved in buffering $K^+$ under pathophysiological conditions.

Astrocyte dysfunction is also involved in other epilepsy syndromes, such as tuberous sclerosis or tumor-associated epilepsy. Tuberous sclerosis complex (TSC) is a common multisystem genetic disorder that frequently involves multiple seizure types. Cortical tubers, a pathologic hallmark of TSC, often represent the site of seizure onset in TSC patients. The cellular features of tubers also include astrocytosis, which indicates that glial dysfunction can be involved in epileptogenesis in TSC. In a mouse model of TSC, the conditional inactivation of the Tsc1 gene in glia (Tsc1GFAPCKO mice) combined with patch-clamp measurements and Western blot analyses revealed that Kir channel function is reduced in astrocytes from these Tsc1GFAPCKO mice both in primary astrocytic cultures and in hippocampal slices *in situ*. Cultured Tsc1-deficient astrocytes exhibited a decreased expression of specific Kir channel protein subunits, Kir2.1 and Kir6.1, and the mRNA expression of these Kir subunits was also reduced in astrocytes from the neocortex. Thus, impaired extracellular $K^+$ uptake by astrocytes through Kir channels may contribute to neuronal hyperexcitability and epileptogenesis in a mouse model of TSC (Jansen et al., 2005). Interestingly, these mice also display a reduced expression of the glutamate transporters GLT1 and GLAST (Wong et al., 2003) and thus impaired glutamate uptake. A typical, epilepsy-associated brain tumor is astrocytoma, in which the involvement of altered $K^+$ homeostasis has been hypothesized in addition to a glutamate hypothesis in tumor-associated epilepsy development. In support of this view, reduced Kir currents and mislocated Kir4.1 channels were described in astrocytoma cells (Bordey and Sontheimer, 1998a; Olsen and Sontheimer, 2004).

Besides Kir channels, attention has recently turned to some members of the $K_{2P}$ channel family, namely TWIK-related acid-sensitive $K^+$ channels 1-3 (TASK 1, 2, 3), especially in regards to their cell-specific expression in different models of epilepsy. In adult seizure-sensitive gerbils, an increased expression of TASK-1 immunoreactivity was detected in hippocampal astrocytes by Kim et al. (2007), indicating their involvement in seizure activity and their possible targeting in treating epilepsy. In a model of pilocarpine-induced epilepsy in rats, Kim et al.(2008) described marked changes in the expression of TASK-1 channels in astrocytes after status epilepticus; these changes are dependent on the astrocyte location within the hippocampal complex. After spontaneous seizure development, a typical reactive gliosis was observed in the dentate gyrus and the CA1 region of the hippocampus; however, only astrocytes in the CA1 region displayed strong immunoreactivity for TASK-1. Additionally, the same group found enhanced TASK-2 immunoreactivity in perivascular regions in the hippocampus, precisely in the endfeet of perivascular astrocytes (Kim et al., 2009). They have suggested that TASK-2 channels might be involved in abnormalities of blood flow regulation or blood-brain barrier impairment after status epilepticus. Recently, in the hippocampus of patients with temporal lobe epilepsy, the augmented immunoreactivity of TASK-1 and TASK-3 was observed predominantly in astrocytes (Kim et al., 2011). Taken together, all of these findings point to the possible role of TASK channels in epilepsy; nevertheless, studies describing functional changes in TASK channels in response to status epilepticus are still lacking.

The role of the astrocytic Kir4.1 channel in seizure generation and progression is further underlined by new findings that show that two similar syndromes characterized by epilepsy, ataxia, sensorineural deafness, mental retardation and renal salt-losing tubulopathy (EAST/SeSAME syndromes) are associated with a mutant KCNJ10 gene encoding the Kir4.1 channels (Bockenhauer et al., 2009; Scholl et al., 2009). Detailed experiments on heterologously expressed Kir4.1 channels or transgenic animals bearing mutations that were found in patients with EAST/SeSAME syndrome have revealed that Kir4.1 channel function is indeed necessary for maintaining $K^+$ homeostasis in the nervous tissue and that its impaired function might lead to the appearance of a seizure-prone phenotype in mice or humans (Sala-Rabanal et al., 2010; Haj-Yasein et al., 2011).

## *Traumatic Brain/Spinal Cord Injuries*

The astrocytic responses to traumatic injury have been extensively studied in many types of CNS injuries, such as a cortical freeze lesion or a cortical stab wound, and they largely depend on the type, extent and location of the injury. The membrane properties of post-traumatic astrocytes have been also studied *in vitro*, in freshly isolated astrocytes from the lesioned cortex (Bevan et al., 1987), in primary cultures of reactive astrocytes isolated from the site of a cortical stab wound (Perillan et al., 1999; Perillan et al., 2000) and in cultured spinal cord astrocytes (MacFarlane and Sontheimer, 1997; Macfarlane and Sontheimer, 1998; MacFarlane and Sontheimer, 2000). Using mechanical scarring of confluent spinal cord astrocytes, an *in vitro* model of CNS injury, MacFarlane and Sontheimer (1997) demonstrated that proliferating astrocytes within the gliotic culture exhibit an approximately threefold reduction in Kir currents, resulting in their marked depolarization, while non-proliferating astrocytes increase their Kir currents. They also showed that the injury-induced electrophysiological changes are rapid, appearing within four hours post-injury, and with respect to Kir currents, not returning to control conductances within 24 hrs. In reactive astrocytes isolated from a gelatin sponge implanted into a cortical stab wound, Perillan et al. (1999) found strong inwardly rectifying K$^+$ currents, which were later identified as Kir2.3 channel subunits (Perillan et al., 2000), thus implying an important functional role for these channels in astrocytes.

a failure of ionic homeostasis in gliotic CNS tissue, followed by abnormal neuronal activity.

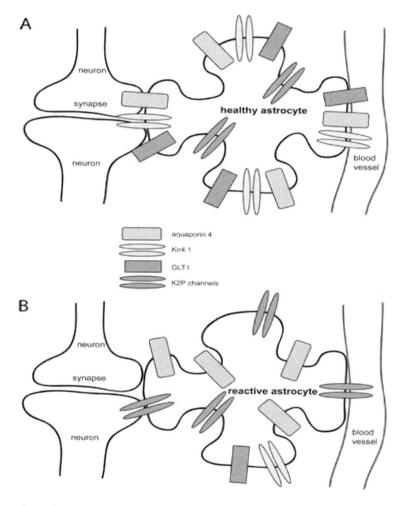

Figure 1. Ion channel expression in "healthy" and reactive astrocytes. A: In healthy nervous tissue, astrocytes express weakly inwardly rectifying K$^+$ channels (Kir4.1) together with aquaporin-4 (AQP4) at the endfeet connecting brain microvessels. Strongly inwardly rectifying Kir2.1 channels and glutamate transporters (GLT1) are predominantly expressed at the endfeet surrounding neuronal synapses. Moreover, astrocytes express the two-pore domain K$^+$ channels TREK1 and TWIK1. B: Reactive astrocytes display a strong down-regulation of Kir4.1 and GLT1 expression and a mislocation of AQP4 channels. On the other hand, they seem to increase their expression of other K$^+$ channels, such as TREK1 and 2.

Since many pathological states are accompanied by an increase in extracellular potassium ($[K^+]_e$), an early event leading to the activation of astrocytes and glial scar formation, several studies have examined the astrocyte membrane properties and cell volume regulation of astrocytes after exposure to high $K^+$ *in situ* (Anderova et al., 2001; Vargova et al., 2001; Neprasova et al., 2007). In an acute model of spinal cord injury, Neprasova et al. (2007) showed that high $[K^+]_e$ does not lead to changes in the Kir current amplitude of passive astrocytes; however, such elevated $K^+$ affects the ability of astrocytes to regulate their volume.

Using an *in vivo* model of brain injury, an increase in $K^+$ inward conductance was found in non-proliferating astrocytes in the hyperexcitable zone that surrounded the core of a neonatal cortical freeze lesion, but proliferating astrocytes showed reduced Kir currents (Bordey et al., 2000; Bordey et al., 2001). A decrease in Kir conductance in reactive glia was also reported following a fluid percussion injury (D'Ambrosio et al., 1999; Schroder et al., 1999) or a cortical stab wound (Anderova et al., 2004). We have described two electrophysiologically, immunohistochemically and morphologically distinct types of hypertrophied astrocytes at the site of a stab wound, depending on the distance from the lesion, which might have different functions in ionic homeostasis. Similarly, in a crush spinal cord injury, Olsen and colleagues have demonstrated that the expression of both Kir4.1 channels and GLT-1 is reduced by ~80% seven days post-injury in adult rats (Olsen et al., 2010). The loss of both membrane proteins extended to spinal segments several millimeters rostral and caudal to the lesion epicenter and persisted 4 weeks post-injury. Taken together, a decrease in Kir currents accompanied by a concomitant increase in outwardly rectifying $K^+$ currents has been clearly shown to be associated with astrocytic proliferation (MacFarlane and Sontheimer, 2000; Bordey et al., 2001; Anderova et al., 2004). Consequently, a decrease in Kir channels may directly impair $K^+$ buffering capacity and thus result in

## *Ischemia*

Accumulating evidence indicates that astrocytes also play an important role in the pathophysiology of cerebral ischemia (Dienel and Hertz, 2005; Nedergaard and Dirnagl, 2005; Anderova et al., 2011). Similar to other CNS injuries, Koller et al. (2000) observed a decrease in Kir currents in glial cells acutely dissociated from the brains of adult rats 3 days after a permanent middle cerebral artery occlusion (MCAO). Recently, we have reported the down-regulation of Kir4.1 channels and the up-regulation of Kir2.1, Kir5.1 and TREK-1 channels in rat hippocampal astrocytes in response to global cerebral ischemia (Pivonkova et al., 2010). Using the patch-clamp technique, we showed that astrocytes in the CA1 region of the hippocampus progressively depolarized starting 3 days after ischemia, which coincided with decreased Kir4.1 protein expression in the gliotic tissue. Other $K^+$ channels described previously in astrocytes, namely Kir2.1, Kir5.1 and TREK1, did not show any changes in their protein content in the ischemic hippocampus; however, based on immunohistochemical analyses, their expression switched from neurons to reactive astrocytes. These findings suggest that after ischemia, astrocytic membrane properties undergo complex alterations that might profoundly influence the maintenance of $K^+$ homeostasis in the damaged tissue. Similar changes in electrophysiological properties and Kir channel expression profile were also reported in radial Muller cells of the ischemic retina, which displayed markedly reduced Kir currents together with increased input resistance and depolarization (Pannicke et al., 2005). In retinal glial cells, proliferative gliosis caused the mislocation of Kir4.1 and Kir2.1 followed by the inactivation of Kir currents (Ulbricht et al., 2008), and ischemia led to decreased Kir4.1 protein expression after 7 days of reperfusion (Iandiev et al., 2006).

Within the $K_{2P}$ channel family, TREK-1,2 channels, which are regulated by polyunsaturated fatty acids, intracellular acidosis and cell swelling (conditions typical of ischemia), have received most of the attention. Initial studies have examined the alterations in the mRNA levels of TREK-2 in response to *in vivo* experimental ischemia in rats. Li et al. (2005) found increased expression of TREK-2 mRNA in the cortex and hippocampus in a model of acute cerebral ischemia, while Xu et al. (2004) found no changes in either region after permanent bilateral carotid artery ligation. Nevertheless, these studies did not differentiate between astrocytic or neuronal TREK-2 mRNA levels. Recently, Kucheryavykh et al. (2009) have demonstrated that under anoxic/hypoglycemic conditions, TREK-2 protein levels as well as TREK-2-like conductance are increased in cultured astrocytes and that TREK-2 channels contribute to glutamate clearance, possibly by maintaining the RMP and astrocyte functions under ischemic conditions by increasing TREK-2 expression. Recently, Zhou et al. (2009) and Chu et al. (2010) showed that mature hipppocampal astrocytes express functional TREK-1 channels, which significantly contribute to passive conductance and help to set the negative RMP essential for the optimal operation of some astrocytic homeostatic functions. The importance of TREK-1 channels in the pathophysiology of cerebral ischemia was pointed out in the recent work of Minghuan Wang and colleagues (Wang et al., 2011). They have observed a significant increase in TREK-1 expression in astrocytes in response to MCAO-induced focal ischemia coinciding with reactive astrogliosis in the cortex and hippocampus. Moreover, they described TREK-1 expression in cultured cortical astrocytes, in which the TREK-1 inhibitor quinine inhibited the proliferation of astrocytes exposed to hypoxia. Their data provides evidence that astrocytic TREK-1 is involved in ischemia pathophysiology.

### *Other Pathological States in the CNS*

Gene expression profiling in astrocytes from hyperammonemic mice revealed the decreased mRNA expression of both Kir4.1 and Kir5.1 channels together with a decreased expression of AQP4 and Cx43 (Lichter-Konecki et al., 2008). More recently, Obara-Michlewska et al. (2011) showed that the hyperammonemia-induced down-regulation of Kir4.1 in astrocytes might result from their higher exposure to glutamate.

# Conclusion

The available data provide strong evidence for the down-regulation of Kir4.1 channel expression in astrocytes, accompanied by functional impairment, after many kinds of acute and chronic CNS injuries. The decrease of Kir4.1 channel expression in reactive astrocytes leads to impaired $K^+$ buffering capacity of the astrocytic syncytium, and it is accompanied by the down-regulation or mislocation of astrocytic membrane proteins, namely aquaporins and glutamate transporters that participate in maintaining water and glutamate homeostasis (Figure 1). On the other hand, the exact cause of Kir4.1 channel down-regulation still remains elusive, and we can only hypothesize that this might be secondarily evoked by a chronic lack of functional neurons and/or prolonged inflammation, at least in some diseases. Nevertheless, whether the down-regulation of Kir4.1 channels is simply a consequence of disease progression or the actual cause of some CNS disorders remains to be elucidated. Taken together, all findings clearly demonstrate that astrocytes undergo profound changes with respect to their $K^+$ channel expression and function after many kinds of CNS injuries and indicate that Kir4.1 channels are an important player in CNS pathologies and a possible target for therapeutic intervention. In addition, the decrease in Kir4.1 channel expression seems to be compensated for by the increased expression of other $K^+$ channels such as other Kir channels (namely Kir2.1) or $K_{2P}$ channels (TREK or TASK), indicating their importance in the progression of CNS diseases and opening new possibilities for therapeutic approaches to affect astrocytic functions in CNS disorders.

## References

Amiry-Moghaddam, M., et al., 2003. Delayed $K^+$ clearance associated with aquaporin-4 mislocalization: phenotypic defects in brains of alpha-syntrophin-null mice. *Proc Natl Acad Sci USA*. 100, 13615-20.

Anderova, M., et al., 2001. Effect of elevated $K(^+)$, hypotonic stress and cortical spreading depression on astrocyte swelling in GFAP-deficient mice. *Glia*. 35, 189-203.

Anderova, M., et al., 2004. Voltage-dependent potassium currents in hypertrophied rat astrocytes after a cortical stab wound. *Glia*. 48, 311-26.

Anderova, M., et al., 2011. Cell death/proliferation and alterations in glial morphology contribute to changes in diffusivity in the rat hippocampus after hypoxia-ischemia. *J Cereb Blood Flow Metab*. 31, 894-907.

Ballanyi, K., Grafe, P., Bruggencate, G., 1987. Ion activities and potassium uptake mechanisms of glial cells in guinea-pig olfactory cortex slices. *J Physiol*. 382, 159-74.

Bevan, S., et al., 1987. Voltage gated ionic channels in rat cultured astrocytes, reactive astrocytes and an astrocyte-oligodendrocyte progenitor cell. *J Physiol* (Paris). 82, 327-35.

Bichet, D., Haass, F.A., Jan, L.Y., 2003. Merging functional studies with structures of inward-rectifier $K(^+)$ channels. *Nat Rev Neurosci*. 4, 957-67.

Bockenhauer, D., et al., 2009. Epilepsy, ataxia, sensorineural deafness, tubulopathy and KCNJ10 mutations. *N Engl J Med*. 360, 1960-70.

Bordey, A., Sontheimer, H., 1998a. Electrophysiological properties of human astrocytic tumor cells In situ: enigma of spiking glial cells. *J Neurophysiol*. 79, 2782-93.

Bordey, A., Sontheimer, H., 1998b. Properties of human glial cells associated with epileptic seizure foci. *Epilepsy Res*. 32, 286-303.

Bordey, A., Hablitz, J.J., Sontheimer, H., 2000. Reactive astrocytes show enhanced inwardly rectifying $K^+$ currents in situ. *Neuroreport*. 11, 3151-5.

Bordey, A., et al., 2001. Electrophysiological characteristics of reactive astrocytes in experimental cortical dysplasia. *J Neurophysiol*. 85, 1719-31.

Butt, A.M., Kalsi, A., 2006. Inwardly rectifying potassium channels (Kir) in central nervous system glia: a special role for Kir4.1 in glial functions. *J Cell Mol Med*. 10, 33-44.

Chever, O., et al., 2010. Implication of Kir4.1 channel in excess potassium clearance: an in vivo study on anesthetized glial-conditional Kir4.1 knock-out mice. *J Neurosci*. 30, 15769-77.

Chu, K.C., et al., 2010. Functional identification of an outwardly rectifying pH- and anesthetic-sensitive leak K($^+$) conductance in hippocampal astrocytes. *Eur J Neurosci*. 32, 725-35.

Cornell-Bell, A.H., Finkbeiner, S.M., 1991. Ca$^{2+}$ waves in astrocytes. *Cell Calcium*. 12, 185-204.

Cui, N., et al., 2001. Modulation of the heteromeric Kir4.1-Kir5.1 channels by P(CO(2)) at physiological levels. *J Cell Physiol*. 189, 229-36.

D'Ambrosio, R., et al., 1998. Functional specialization and topographic segregation of hippocampal astrocytes. *J Neurosci*. 18, 4425-38.

D'Ambrosio, R., et al., 1999. Impaired K($^+$) homeostasis and altered electrophysiological properties of post-traumatic hippocampal glia. *J Neurosci*. 19, 8152-62.

D'Ambrosio, R., Gordon, D.S., Winn, H.R., 2002. Differential role of KIR channel and Na($^+$)/K($^+$)-pump in the regulation of extracellular K($^+$) in rat hippocampus. *J Neurophysiol*. 87, 87-102.

Dienel, G.A., Hertz, L., 2005. Astrocytic contributions to bioenergetics of cerebral ischemia. *Glia*. 50, 362-88.

Djukic, B., et al., 2007. Conditional knock-out of Kir4.1 leads to glial membrane depolarization, inhibition of potassium and glutamate uptake and enhanced short-term synaptic potentiation. *J Neurosci*. 27, 11354-65.

Doetsch, F., et al., 1999. Subventricular zone astrocytes are neural stem cells in the adult mammalian brain. *Cell*. 97, 703-16.

Ducret, T., Vacher, A.M., Vacher, P., 2003. Voltage-dependent ionic conductances in the human malignant astrocytoma cell line U87-MG. *Mol Membr Biol*. 20, 329-43.

Fawcett, J.W., Asher, R.A., 1999. The glial scar and central nervous system repair. *Brain Res Bull*. 49, 377-91.

Ferroni, S., et al., 2003. Arachidonic acid activates an open rectifier potassium channel in cultured rat cortical astrocytes. *J Neurosci Res*. 72, 363-72.

Gnatenco, C., et al., 2002. Functional expression of TREK-2 K$^+$ channel in cultured rat brain astrocytes. *Brain Res*. 931, 56-67.

Goldstein, S.A., et al., 2001. Potassium leak channels and the KCNK family of two-P-domain subunits. *Nat Rev Neurosci*. 2, 175-84.

Gordon, G.R., Mulligan, S. J., MacVicar, B. A., 2007. Astrocyte control of the cerebro-vasculature. *Glia*. 55, 1214-21.

Haj-Yasein, N.N., et al., 2011. Evidence that compromised K($^+$) spatial buffering contributes to the epileptogenic effect of mutations in the human Kir4.1 gene (KCNJ10). *Glia*. 59, 1635-42.

Haydon, P.G., 2001. GLIA: listening and talking to the synapse. *Nat Rev Neurosci*. 2, 185-93.

Heinemann, U., Lux, H.D., 1977. Ceiling of stimulus induced rises in extracellular potassium concentration in the cerebral cortex of cat. *Brain Res*. 120, 231-49.

Hibino, H., et al., 2004. Differential assembly of inwardly rectifying K$^+$ channel subunits, Kir4.1 and Kir5.1, in brain astrocytes. *J Biol Chem*. 279, 44065-73.

Hibino, H., et al., 2010. Inwardly rectifying potassium channels: their structure, function and physiological roles. *Physiol Rev*. 90, 291-366.

Hinterkeuser, S., et al., 2000. Astrocytes in the hippocampus of patients with temporal lobe epilepsy display changes in potassium conductances. *Eur J Neurosci.* 12, 2087-96.

Homola, A., et al., 2006. Changes in diffusion parameters, energy-related metabolites and glutamate in the rat cortex after transient hypoxia/ischemia. *Neurosci Lett.* 404, 137-42.

Honore, E., 2007. The neuronal background K2P channels: focus on TREK1. *Nat Rev Neurosci.* 8, 251-61.

Iandiev, I., et al., 2006. Differential regulation of Kir4.1 and Kir2.1 expression in the ischemic rat retina. *Neurosci Lett.* 396, 97-101.

Inyushin, M., et al., 2010. Potassium channel activity and glutamate uptake are impaired in astrocytes of seizure-susceptible DBA/2 mice. *Epilepsia.* 51, 1707-13.

Jalonen, T.O., Charniga, C.J., Wielt, D.B., 1997. beta-Amyloid peptide-induced morphological changes coincide with increased $K^+$ and Cl- channel activity in rat cortical astrocytes. *Brain Res.* 746, 85-97.

Janigro, D., et al., 1997. Reduction of $K^+$ uptake in glia prevents long-term depression maintenance and causes epileptiform activity. *J Neurosci.* 17, 2813-24.

Jansen, L.A., et al., 2005. Epileptogenesis and reduced inward rectifier potassium current in tuberous sclerosis complex-1-deficient astrocytes. *Epilepsia.* 46, 1871-80.

Kaiser, M., et al., 2006. Progressive loss of a glial potassium channel (KCNJ10) in the spinal cord of the SOD1 (G93A) transgenic mouse model of amyotrophic lateral sclerosis. *J Neurochem.* 99, 900-12.

Kang, S.J., et al., 2008. Expression of Kir2.1 channels in astrocytes under pathophysiological conditions. *Mol Cells.* 25, 124-30.

Kim, D., et al., 2009. Heteromeric TASK-1/TASK-3 is the major oxygen-sensitive background $K^+$ channel in rat carotid body glomus cells. *J Physiol.* 587, 2963-75.

Kim, D.S., et al., 2007. Up-regulated astroglial TWIK-related acid-sensitive $K^+$ channel-1 (TASK-1) in the hippocampus of seizure-sensitive gerbils: a target of anti-epileptic drugs. *Brain Res.* 1185, 346-58.

Kim, J.E., et al., 2008. Region-specific alterations in astroglial TWIK-related acid-sensitive $K^+$-1 channel immunoreactivity in the rat hippocampal complex following pilocarpine-induced status epilepticus. *J Comp Neurol.* 510, 463-74.

Kim, J.E., et al., 2011. Changes in TWIK-related Acid Sensitive $K(^+)$-1 and -3 Channel Expressions from Neurons to Glia in the Hippocampus of Temporal Lobe Epilepsy Patients and Experimental Animal Model. *Neurochem Res.*

Kofuji, P., et al., 2000. Genetic inactivation of an inwardly rectifying potassium channel (Kir4.1 subunit) in mice: phenotypic impact in retina. *J Neurosci.* 20, 5733-40.

Kofuji, P., et al., 2002. Kir potassium channel subunit expression in retinal glial cells: implications for spatial potassium buffering. *Glia.* 39, 292-303.

Kofuji, P., Newman, E.A., 2004. Potassium buffering in the central nervous system. *Neuroscience.* 129, 1045-56.

Koller, H., et al., 2000. Time course of inwardly rectifying $K(^+)$ current reduction in glial cells surrounding ischemic brain lesions. *Brain Res.* 872, 194-8.

Kubo, Y., et al., 2005. International Union of Pharmacology. LIV. Nomenclature and molecular relationships of inwardly rectifying potassium channels. *Pharmacol Rev.* 57, 509-26.

Kucheryavykh, L.Y., et al., 2009. Ischemia Increases TREK-2 Channel Expression in Astrocytes: Relevance to Glutamate Clearance. *Open Neurosci J.* 3, 40-47.

Kucheryavykh, Y.V., et al., 2007. Down-regulation of Kir4.1 inward rectifying potassium channel subunits by RNAi impairs potassium transfer and glutamate uptake by cultured cortical astrocytes. *Glia.* 55, 274-81.

Kuffler, S.W., Nicholls, J.G., Orkand, R.K., 1966. Physiological properties of glial cells in the central nervous system of amphibia. *J Neurophysiol.* 29, 768-87.

Kunzelmann, K., 2005. Ion channels and cancer. *J Membr Biol.* 205, 159-73.

Li, Z.B., et al., 2005. Enhanced expressions of arachidonic acid-sensitive tandem-pore domain potassium channels in rat experimental acute cerebral ischemia. *Biochem Biophys Res Commun.* 327, 1163-9.

Lichter-Konecki, U., et al., 2008. Gene expression profiling of astrocytes from hyper-ammonemic mice reveals altered pathways for water and potassium homeostasis in vivo. *Glia.* 56, 365-77.

MacFarlane, S.N., Sontheimer, H., 1997. Electrophysiological changes that accompany reactive gliosis in vitro. *J Neurosci.* 17, 7316-29.

Macfarlane, S.N., Sontheimer, H., 1998. Spinal cord astrocytes display a switch from TTX-sensitive to TTX-resistant sodium currents after injury-induced gliosis in vitro. *J Neurophysiol.* 79, 2222-6.

MacFarlane, S.N., Sontheimer, H., 2000. Changes in ion channel expression accompany cell cycle progression of spinal cord astrocytes. *Glia.* 30, 39-48.

Meeks, J.P., Mennerick, S., 2007. Astrocyte membrane responses and potassium accumulation during neuronal activity. *Hippocampus.* 17, 1100-8.

Menn, B., et al., 2006. Origin of oligodendrocytes in the subventricular zone of the adult brain. *J Neurosci.* 26, 7907-18.

Mishima, T., Hirase, H., 2010. In vivo intracellular recording suggests that gray matter astrocytes in mature cerebral cortex and hippocampus are electrophysiologically homogeneous. *J Neurosci.* 30, 3093-100.

Muller, M., Somjen, G.G., 2000. $Na^{+}$ and $K^{+}$ concentrations, extra- and intracellular voltages, and the effect of TTX in hypoxic rat hippocampal slices. *J Neurophysiol.* 83, 735-45.

Nagelhus, E.A., et al., 1999. Immunogold evidence suggests that coupling of $K^+$ siphoning and water transport in rat retinal Muller cells is mediated by a co-enrichment of Kir4.1 and AQP4 in specific membrane domains. *Glia.* 26, 47-54.

Nagelhus, E.A., Mathiisen, T.M., Ottersen, O.P., 2004. Aquaporin-4 in the central nervous system: cellular and subcellular distribution and coexpression with KIR4.1. *Neuroscience.* 129, 905-13.

Nedergaard, M., Ransom, B., Goldman, S.A., 2003. New roles for astrocytes: redefining the functional architecture of the brain. *Trends Neurosci.* 26, 523-30.

Nedergaard, M., Dirnagl, U., 2005. Role of glial cells in cerebral ischemia. *Glia.* 50, 281-6.

Neprasova, H., et al., 2007. High extracellular K(+) evokes changes in voltage-dependent K(+) and Na (+) currents and volume regulation in astrocytes. *Pflugers Arch.* 453, 839-49.

Neusch, C., et al., 2006. Lack of the Kir4.1 channel subunit abolishes $K^+$ buffering properties of astrocytes in the ventral respiratory group: impact on extracellular $K^+$ regulation. *J Neurophysiol.* 95, 1843-52.

Newman, E.A., Frambach, D.A., Odette, L.L., 1984. Control of extracellular potassium levels by retinal glial cell $K^+$ siphoning. *Science.* 225, 1174-5.

Newman, E.A., 1986. High potassium conductance in astrocyte endfeet. *Science.* 233, 453-4.

Obara-Michlewska, M., et al., 2011. Down-regulation of Kir4.1 in the cerebral cortex of rats with liver failure and in cultured astrocytes treated with glutamine: Implications for astrocytic dysfunction in hepatic encephalopathy. *J Neurosci Res.*

Olabarria, M., et al., 2010. Concomitant astroglial atrophy and astrogliosis in a triple transgenic animal model of Alzheimer's disease. *Glia.* 58, 831-8.

Olsen, M.L., Sontheimer, H., 2004. Mislocalization of Kir channels in malignant glia. *Glia.* 46, 63-73.

Olsen, M.L., Sontheimer, H., 2008. Functional implications for Kir4.1 channels in glial biology: from $K^+$ buffering to cell differentiation. *J Neurochem.* 107, 589-601.

Olsen, M.L., et al., 2010. Spinal cord injury causes a wide-spread, persistent loss of Kir4.1 and glutamate transporter 1: benefit of 17 beta-oestradiol treatment. *Brain.* 133, 1013-25.

Orkand, R.K., Nicholls, J.G., Kuffler, S.W., 1966. Effect of nerve impulses on the membrane potential of glial cells in the central nervous system of amphibia. *J Neurophysiol.* 29, 788-806.

Orkand, R.K., 1986. Glial-interstitial fluid exchange. *Ann N Y Acad Sci.* 481, 269-72.

Pannicke, T., et al., 2005. Altered membrane physiology in Muller glial cells after transient ischemia of the rat retina. *Glia.* 50, 1-11.

Pasler, D., Gabriel, S., Heinemann, U., 2007. Two-pore-domain potassium channels contribute to neuronal potassium release and glial potassium buffering in the rat hippocampus. *Brain Res.* 1173, 14-26.

Perillan, P.R., Li, X., Simard, J.M., 1999. K(+) inward rectifier currents in reactive astrocytes from adult rat brain. *Glia.* 27, 213-25.

Perillan, P.R., et al., 2000. Inward rectifier K(+) channel Kir2.3 (IRK3) in reactive astrocytes from adult rat brain. *Glia.* 31, 181-92.

Peters, O., et al., 2009. Astrocyte function is modified by Alzheimer's disease-like pathology in aged mice. *J Alzheimers Dis.* 18, 177-89.

Pivonkova, H., et al., 2010. Impact of global cerebral ischemia on $K^+$ channel expression and membrane properties of glial cells in the rat hippocampus. *Neurochem Int.* 57, 783-94.

Poopalasundaram, S., et al., 2000. Glial heterogeneity in expression of the inwardly rectifying K(+) channel, Kir4.1, in adult rat CNS. *Glia.* 30, 362-72.

Ransom, C.B., Sontheimer, H., 1995. Biophysical and pharmacological characterization of inwardly rectifying $K^+$ currents in rat spinal cord astrocytes. *J Neurophysiol.* 73, 333-46.

Ransom, C.B., Sontheimer, H., 2001. BK channels in human glioma cells. *J Neurophysiol.* 85, 790-803.

Rothstein, J.D., et al., 1996. Knockout of glutamate transporters reveals a major role for astroglial transport in excitotoxicity and clearance of glutamate. *Neuron.* 16, 675-86.

Rusznak, Z., et al., 2004. Differential distribution of TASK-1, TASK-2 and TASK-3 immunoreactivities in the rat and human cerebellum. *Cell Mol Life Sci.* 61, 1532-42.

Sala-Rabanal, M., et al., 2010. Molecular mechanisms of EAST/SeSAME syndrome mutations in Kir4.1 (KCNJ10). *J Biol Chem.* 12, 36040-8. .

Scholl, U.I., et al., 2009. Seizures, sensorineural deafness, ataxia, mental retardation and electrolyte imbalance (SeSAME syndrome) caused by mutations in KCNJ10. *Proc Natl Acad Sci USA.* 106, 5842-7.

Schroder, W., et al., 1999. Lesion-induced changes of electrophysiological properties in astrocytes of the rat dentate gyrus. *Glia.* 28, 166-74.

Schroder, W., et al., 2000. Functional and molecular properties of human astrocytes in acute hippocampal slices obtained from patients with temporal lobe epilepsy. *Epilepsia.* 41 Suppl 6, S181-4.

Seifert, G., et al., 2009. Analysis of astroglial $K^+$ channel expression in the developing hippocampus reveals a predominant role of the Kir4.1 subunit. *J Neurosci.* 29, 7474-88.

Seri, B., et al., 2004. Cell types, lineage and architecture of the germinal zone in the adult dentate gyrus. *J Comp Neurol.* 478, 359-78.

Stewart, T.H., et al., 2010. Chronic dysfunction of astrocytic inwardly rectifying $K^+$ channels specific to the neocortical epileptic focus after fluid percussion injury in the rat. *J Neurophysiol.* 104, 3345-60.

Swanson, R.A., Ying, W., Kauppinen, T. M., 2004. Astrocyte influences on ischemic neuronal death. *Curr Mol Med.* 4, 193-205.

Tan, G., Sun, S.Q., Yuan, D.L., 2008. Expression of Kir4.1 in human astrocytic tumors: correlation with pathologic grade. *Biochem Biophys Res Commun.* 367, 743-7.

Tanaka, K., et al., 1997. Epilepsy and exacerbation of brain injury in mice lacking the glutamate transporter GLT-1. *Science.* 276, 1699-702.

Theis, M., et al., 2003. Accelerated hippocampal spreading depression and enhanced locomotory activity in mice with astrocyte-directed inactivation of connexin43. *J Neurosci.* 23, 766-76.

Trachtenberg, M.C., Pollen, D.A., 1970. Neuroglia: biophysical properties and physiologic function. *Science.* 167, 1248-52.

Ulbricht, E., et al., 2008. Proliferative gliosis causes mislocation and inactivation of inwardly rectifying $K(^+)$ (Kir) channels in rabbit retinal glial cells. *Exp Eye Res.* 86, 305-13.

Vargova, L., et al., 2001. Effect of osmotic stress on potassium accumulation around glial cells and extracellular space volume in rat spinal cord slices. *J Neurosci Res.* 65, 129-38.

Verkman, A.S., 2005. More than just water channels: unexpected cellular roles of aquaporins. *J Cell Sci.* 118, 3225-32.

Wallraff, A., et al., 2006. The impact of astrocytic gap junctional coupling on potassium buffering in the hippocampus. *J Neurosci.* 26, 5438-47.

Walz, W., 2000. Role of astrocytes in the clearance of excess extracellular potassium. *Neurochem Int.* 36, 291-300.

Wang, D.D., Bordey, A., 2008. The astrocyte odyssey. *Prog Neurobiol.* 86, 342-67.

Wang, M., et al., 2011. Changes in Lipid-Sensitive Two-Pore Domain Potassium Channel TREK-1 Expression and Its Involvement in Astrogliosis Following Cerebral Ischemia in Rats. *J Mol Neurosci.*

Warth, A., Mittelbronn, M., Wolburg, H., 2005. Redistribution of the water channel protein aquaporin-4 and the $K^+$ channel protein Kir4.1 differs in low- and high-grade human brain tumors. *Acta Neuropathol.* 109, 418-26.

Wilcock, D.M., Vitek, M.P., Colton, C.A., 2009. Vascular amyloid alters astrocytic water and potassium channels in mouse models and humans with Alzheimer's disease. *Neuroscience.* 159, 1055-69.

Wong, M., et al., 2003. Impaired glial glutamate transport in a mouse tuberous sclerosis epilepsy model. *Ann Neurol.* 54, 251-6.

Xu, X., Pan, Y., Wang, X., 2004. Alterations in the expression of lipid and mechano-gated two-pore domain potassium channel genes in rat brain following chronic cerebral ischemia. *Brain Res Mol Brain Res.* 120, 205-9.

Zhou, M., et al., 2009. TWIK-1 and TREK-1 are potassium channels contributing significantly to astrocyte passive conductance in rat hippocampal slices. *J Neurosci.* 29, 8551-64.

*Chapter III*

# The Phosphoinositides Signal Transduction Pathway in Astrocytes

*Vincenza Rita Lo Vasco*[*]
Department Organi di Senso, Policlinico Umberto I, Faculty
of Medicine and Odontoiatry, Sapienza University of Rome
Viale del Policlinico, Rome, Italy

## Abstract

Signal transduction from plasma membrane to cell nucleus is a complex process depending on various components including lipid signaling molecules. Phosphoinositides (PI) constitute an important signaling system. Enzymes related to the PI signal transduction pathway may act at cell periphery, plasma membrane or nuclear level. The PI cycle was also hypothesized to be involved in neuronal as well as glial activities. Many evidences support the hypothesis that the PI cycle is involved in astrocytes activation during the neurodegeneration process. Phosphoinositide-specific phospholipase C (PI-PLC) family of enzymes is crucial in PI signaling system. In fact, PI-PLC enzymes regulate the spatial and temporal balance of PI. Thirteen mammalian PI-PLC isoforms were identified, divided into six sub-families on the basis of amino acid sequence, domain structure and mechanism of recruitment in response to activated receptors: β (1–4), γ (1, 2), δ (1, 3, 4), ε (1), ζ (1), and η (1-2). Different expression of the isoforms was described in pathological cells with respect to the corresponding normal counterparts. The expression panel of PI-PLC isoforms varies under different conditions, such as tumoral progression or inflammatory activation, with respect to the quiescent astrocytes counterpart. These observations suggest that in the nervous system the fine regulation of PI-PLC isoforms play a role in the activation of the glia and in the inflammation processes.

---

[*] Mail address: ritalovasco@hotmail.it; vincenzarita.lovasco@uniroma1.it; Phone +39 06 4997 6817; Fax +39 06 4997 6814.

# Introduction

Cells own complex systems enabling their communication, by means of a number of signaling molecules such as small peptides, proteins, aminoacids, nucleotides, steroids, retinoids, fatty acids and derivatives, gases including nitric oxide (NO) and carbon monoxide. In response to specific stimuli, every cell modulates its activity. Accordingly to the intracellular machinery, the cells receive signals, integrate and properly respond. That results in differentiation, proliferation, stand by or apoptosis depending on the set of signals that, in the presence of specific receptors, the cell is tuned to catch [1]. Thanks to this complex organization, cells adapt to environmental changes.

In the nervous system, the information is transmitted at synapses among neurons. Recent advances, improving the knowledge of astrocyte functions, modified the neuron centric view. The synaptic transmission involves the release of neurotransmitters at individual synapses in response to a single action potential. The tripartite synapse hypothesis proposes that glial cells represent functional components of synapses [2].

Astrocytes directly or indirectly control a number of functions, such as neurotransmitter uptake and recycling, neurometabolism and blood flow regulation. In contrast to previous notions, astrocytes are known to possess their own forms of signaling, as recently highlighted by fuctional imaging methods, such as magnetic resonance (fMRI) and positron emission tomography (PET).

Astrocytes contribute to the processing of information by detecting the neurotransmitters which were released during the neuronal activity [3-4] and, in turn, by modulating the synaptic transmission [3-7].

Astrocytes modulate the activity of neuronal networks upon sustained and intense synaptic activity. In fact, astrocytes release neuroactive substances, termed gliotransmitters, such as purines, D-serine, and glutamate [8-9]. Astrocyte activation occurs at functional compartments found along the astrocytic processes. In response to activation, astrocytes increase the basal synaptic transmission, as suggested by the blockade of their activity obtained by means of calcium chelators [7].

# The Role of Calcium in Astrocytes

Calcium is a crucial mediator in a number of activities, both in cells and tissues. The regulation of synapses by astrocytes involves the mobilization of intracellular calcium and results from receptor activation, with special regard to group I metabotropic glutamatergic receptors (mGluR) [3; 10-11].

Calcium responses may be evoked in distinct areas of Bergmann glial cells [12]. Rapid detection of glutamatergic transmission by astrocytes occurs via glutamate transporter currents generated by synaptic release of glutamate [13]. The synaptic modulation is driven by receptor activation through calcium dependent mechanisms, indicating that astrocytes possess high levels of sensitivity to neurotransmitters. The balanced modulation of activities requires that astrocytes contribute to increase or decrease the basal synaptic transmission. The local modulation might be extended to the whole astrocyte by the propagation of calcium signals along the astrocytic processes.

Glutamatergic and cholinergic pathways in the CA1 region of hippocampus might influence each other, modulating the amplitude of the astrocytic calcium signal and its propagation from the processes to the soma [6]. The astrocytes then switch from local integration to global level, acting as synaptic integrators in the neural network. Probably, different sets of mechanisms and calcium sensitivity are involved. Therefore, in the astrocytes pattern, temporal profile, and magnitude of the calcium changes are critical for different regulatory functions [5]. The activities of the astrocytes are influenced by the types of activated receptors. Local calcium responses are mediated by mGluR5, whereas glutamatergic receptors (mGluR and NMDA receptors) are involved in astrocyte excitability and modulation [8].

The detection of local and rapid basal synaptic transmission suggests that astrocytes discriminate at multiple levels of communication, from basal synaptic activity at unitary synapses up to complex patterns of multisynaptic network interactions [3-7]. Thus, astrocytes are able to decode the pattern of synaptic activity and, in turn, to differentially modulate the output of the synaptic transmission. In fact, specific patterns of calcium activities induce distinct forms of synaptic plasticity at the neuromuscular junction [14].

A number of studies attempted to identify the metabolic processes occurring in astrocytes during the neural signaling. The neural metabolism is mainly oxidative. Glucose is oxidatively converted into more useful forms of energy, such as adenosine triphosphate (ATP). However, cerebral glucose consumption exceeds the oxygen utilization during brain activity [15-16], suggesting that the metabolic needs are also partially covered non-oxidatively.

This observation, initially controversial [17], was corroborated by descriptions of activity-related increases of the metabolic end-product of glycolysis, namely the cerebral lactate [18]. Under aerobic conditions, the production of extracellular lactate increases with glucose availability in cultured astrocytes, but not in cultured neurons. Under anaerobic conditions, the lactate efflux from both neurons and astrocytes increases [19]. Increased glutamate uptake stimulates the conversion of glucose to lactate in cultured astrocytes [20], suggesting that lactate from astrocytic glycolysis is used as an energy substrate to fuel increasing neuronal oxidative metabolism [20].

Synaptic terminals represent the most energy-demanding sites in nervous tissue [21-22].

Neural processes are accompanied by local vascular changes [23], although the regulation of this process remains to be fully elucidated. Blood delivery increases with the metabolic demand. The blood flow, as well as the glucose consumption, increases more than oxygen utilization. Both oxidative and non-oxidative processes follow increased metabolic requirements.

The astrocytes mediate the vascular changes observed during the neural signaling. Recent advances indicated that astrocytes control local cerebrovascular microcirculation [24], influencing the intracellular calcium fluxes [5; 25]. Measures of the latency of calcium responses confirmed that stimulus-induced astrocyte activity is rapidly invoked (in a few seconds) in vivo.

As a matter of fact, astrocytes undergo highly tuned intracellular calcium fluxes [24]. Therefore, great interest was paid to the signaling of calcium. Recent studies [26-28] suggested a role for PI transduction pathway in the fine regulation of calcium levels in astrocytes related to neural activity.

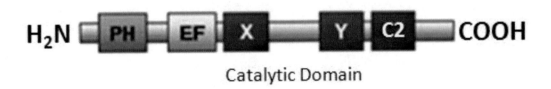

Figure 1. PI-PLC general structure. Domains are indicated (see the text).

## Phosphoinositide Signal Transduction System

PI signal transduction pathway stimulated the fervour of researchers inasmuch potentially involved in a growing number of diseases. The role for PI in signal transduction was first described in 1953 [29]. Extracellular signals stimulated the incorporation of radioactive phosphate into cell membrane phosphatidylinositol [30].

Later, the existence of a PI cycle in the nucleus, distinguished from the cell membrane inositol cycle, was demonstrated [31].

Phosphoinositide-specific phospholipase C (PI-PLC) enzymes are involved in PI signaling (Figure 1) [32-33].

Accordingly to what is known for hormones, a double response induction exists also for PI-PLC enzymes activities. Direct induction of the transcription of a small number of selected genes (within maximum 1h) (primary response) produces proteins, which in turn activate other genes and produce a delayed (secondary) response (Figure 2).

PI-PLC enzymes seem to be involved in the progression of various tumours [34-35] and in the inflammatory activation of glia [27].

Moreover, the possible role of PI-PLC enzymes in the ethiopathogenesis of mental illnesses, such as major depression [36] and schizophrenia [37-40] was investigated. Such observations indicated that PI-PLC enzymes might be involved in the alteration of neurotransmission. The nature and the meaning of this involvement are still unclear.

## PI Metabolism

The metabolism of PI contributes an important signaling system involved in a variety of cell functions, including hormone secretion, neurotransmitter signal transduction, cell growth, membrane trafficking, ion channel activity, cytoskeleton regulation, cell cycle control and apoptosis [33].

Therefore, the second messenger cascade of PI signaling contributes to the regulation of a variety of biological functions such as cell motility, fertilization and sensory transduction. Analyses of genetically modified mice revealed that PI play fundamental and specific roles in embryonic development and organogenesis [41].

Involvement of PI in cell and tissue polarity regulation was also suggested [42].

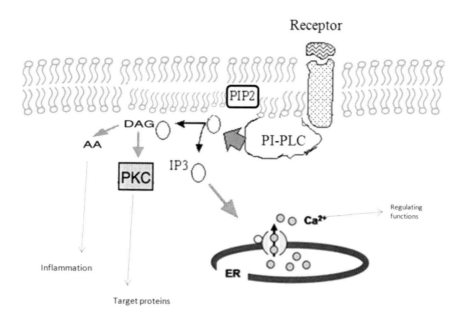

Figure 2. PI-PLC pathway (see the text).

## Table 1. PI-PLC genes localization

| Enzyme | gene | OMIM | gene localization |
|---|---|---|---|
| PI-PLC β1 | PLCB1 | *607120 | 20p12 |
| PI-PLC β2 | PLCB2 | *604114 | 15q15 |
| PI-PLC β3 | PLCB3 | *600230 | 11q13 |
| PI-PLC β4 | PLCB4 | *600810 | 20p12 |
| PI-PLC γ1 | PLCG1 | *172420 | 20q12-q13.1 |
| PI-PLC γ2 | PLCG2 | *600220 | 16q24.1 |
| PI-PLC δ1 | PLCD1 | *602142 | 3p22-p21.3 |
| PI-PLC δ3 | PLCD3 | *608795 | 17q21 |
| PI-PLC δ4 | PLCD4 | *605939 | 2q35 |
| PI-PLC ε | PLCE | *608414 | 10q23 |
| PI-PLC η1 | PLCH1 | *612835 | 3q25.31 |
| PI-PLC η2 | PLCH2 | *612836 | 1p36.32 |
| PI-PLC ζ | PLCZ | *608075 | 12p12.3 |

PI-PLC enzymes (first column, left), corresponding genes (second column), on line Mendelina Inheritance in Man Catalogue (OMIM) number identification (third column) and gene localization on human chromosomes (fourth column, right).

Two phosphorylated derivatives of PI, the phosphatydil inositol phosphate (PIP) and the phosphatydil inositol bisphosphate (PIP2), located mainly in the inner half of the plasma membrane lipid bilayer, are involved in signaling events.

A combination of compartmentalized and temporal changes in the PIP2 or phosphatidyl inositol 3,4,5 trisphosphate (PIP3) levels might elicit different cellular responses, including regulation of gene expression, DNA replication, or chromatin degradation. PIP2 directly regulates a variety of cell functions, including cytoskeletal reorganization, cytokinesis, membrane dynamics, nuclear events and channel activity [33]. Therefore, strict regulation of PIP2 levels is necessary for homeostasis. Many molecules interfere with PI metabolism, such as the PI-PLC family of enzymes [33]. PI-PLC enzymes play a central role by regulating the spatio-temporal balance of PI metabolism. PIP2 is hydrolyzed by means of PI-PLC in response to a wide panel of stimuli, including growth factors (GF), hormones and neurotransmitters, which act on specific receptors localized at the plasma membrane [43].

As a response, after a molecule binds to a G-protein-linked receptor in the plasma membrane (Gq) activates PI-PLC. In less than a second, PI-PLC cleaves the polar head group of PIP2 into IP3 and DAG, both crucial molecules in signal transduction. IP3 is a universal calcium mobilizing. DAG is an activator of several types of effector proteins [33]. Both these second messengers provide a common link from highly specific receptors for hormones, neurotransmitters, antigens, components of the extracellular matrix and GF to downstream intracellular targets [44]. IP3, a small water-soluble molecule, diffuses rapidly to the cytoplasm, where it induces release of calcium from the endoplasmic reticulum binding to IP3-gated calcium-release channels located in the reticulum membrane [33]. On the other hand, DAG exerts two potential signaling roles. First, it can be further cleaved to release arachidonic acid, which either acts as a messenger or is used in the synthesis of eicosanoids. Therefore, DAG is indirectly involved in the inflammatory cascade process [33].

Second, DAG activates the serine/threonine calcium dependent protein kinases C (PKC). The increase of calcium levels moves PKC to translocate from the cytoplasm to the cytoplasmic face of the plasma membrane. The translocation activates PKC enzymes, which regulate the activity of further target proteins by phosphorylation [44] (Figure 2).

## PI-PLC Family of Enzymes

PI-PLC enzymes were classified on the basis of amino acid sequence, domain structure and mechanism of recruitment in response to activated receptors. PI-PLC enzymes are codified by different genes. Gene sequence analyses demonstrated that each isoform has more than one alternative splicing variant, probably having slightly different activity [33] (Table 1).

Thirteen mammalian PI-PLC isoforms were identified, divided into six sub-families: $\beta(1-4)$, $\gamma(1, 2)$, $\delta(1, 3, 4)$, $\epsilon(1)$, $\zeta(1)$, and $\eta(2)$ [33].

Isoforms within the sub-families share sequence similarity, common domain organization, and regulatory mechanism. PI-PLC isozymes contain catalytic X and Y domains as well as various regulatory domains, including the protein kinase C conserved region 2 (C2) domain, EF-hand motif, and pleckstrin homology (PH) domain. The PH domain, of 110 amino acids, binds PI. The X and Y domains fold to form the catalytic site. The X domain (65 aminoacids) binds calcium. The Y domain (115 aminoacids) binds primarily the substrate [33] (Figure 1). Beside the shared core architecture, further domains were described. The PH domain from PI-PLC $\delta 1$ binds $PIP_2$ with high affinity and might be flexibly positioned relative to the other three domains [44]. The central C2 domain interacts with both EF-hands and the catalytic TIM barrel [44]. In PI-PLC $\beta 2$ the PH domain is packed tightly between the EF-hands and TIM barrel resulting in a compact and globular core. It also mediates protein–protein interactions through binding the GTP-bound form of Rac and Cdc42 [44]. Based on these structural insights and domain organization, the EF-hands–C2 domain–

TIM barrel unit probably will be structurally highly similar in all PI-PLC isoforms with the N-terminal PH domain attached either loosely or making different interactions with other domains [44]. In PI-PLC β and η subfamilies unique regions are linked to the C-terminus of the core structure. The structure of the C-terminal extension from PI-PLC β was solved, forming a novel fold composed almost entirely of three long helices forming a coiled-coil [44]. This structure contains elements involved in dimerization and an electrostatically positive surface. The C-terminal extension in PI-PLC ε contains two ubiquitin-like (Ub) folds [44]. The PI-PLC ε RA2 domain can bind Ras GTPases owing to overall positive charge and specific residues involved in Ras-binding. PI-PLC ε also contains a N-terminal cell division control 25 (CDC25) guanine-nucleotide exchange factor (GEF) domain. That domain was predicted to be structurally similar to son of sevenless (SOS), which confers function as an upstream activator of small GTPases [44]. In PI-PLC γ subfamily an insertion (PLCγ-specific array; γSA) is located between X and Y domains [44], a highly structured region. The γSA includes a second, 'split' PH (spPH) domain. Probably, the two parts of the spPH domain form a stable, single domain with a loop incorporating SH domains [44]. PI-PLC ζ lacks the PH domain.

Subtype-specific domains contribute to specific regulatory mechanisms. PI-PLC enzymes cover a broad spectrum of interactions that contribute to membrane recruitment, including binding to PI, interaction with small GTPases from Ras and Rho families or heterotrimeric G protein subunits and recognition of specific sites in tyrosine kinase receptors [33]. Studies distinguished differences in the regulation of PI-PLC γ and of PI-PLC β isoforms by Gα and Gβγ subunits of heterotrimeric G proteins. Further studies of PI-PLC subfamilies, with special regard to PI-PLC ε, revealed a regulatory unique link, thus suggesting a complex interplay between different subfamilies and their regulatory networks [44]. PI-PLC ε is directly regulated by small GTPases from the Ras family and its activity can be stimulated by subunits of heterotrimeric G proteins and small GTPases from the Rho family [44].

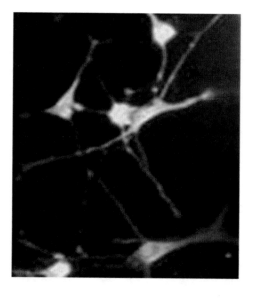

Figure 3. (Continued).

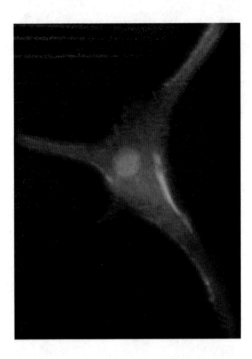

Figure 3. Immunohistochemistry microphotographs. Picture of LPS activated astrocytes observed with fluorescence microscope. (left) 40X: detection of PI-PLC β4 antibody. (right) 100X: detection of PI-PLC δ4 antibody.

The tissue distribution of PI-PLC seems to be strictly specific, suggesting that each isoform bears a unique function in the modulation of physiological responses. PI-PLC isoforms were detected in many tissues, being preferentially expressed in hematopoietic cell lines (PI-PLC β2 and γ2) and in the nervous system (cerebrovisual cortex) (PI-PLC β4). PI-PLC δ1 is widely expressed in many tissues, especially in cultured cells [45-48]. PI-PLC δ3 was identified in a number of histotypes, although at low concentrations [49]. PI-PLC δ4 is expressed in the brain as well as in regenerating tissues [50]. PI-PLC γ1 is expressed in keratinocytes and foetal cartilage [51], mainly in the cytoplasm [52-53]. PI-PLC ε occurs in a number of tissues [54]. PI-PLC ζ was identified exclusively in spermatid cells [55]. PI-PLC η isoforms, the most recently identified, seemed to be highly expressed in neuron-enriched brain regions [33]. Recent evidences indicated that PI-PLC η isoforms are expressed in human umbilical vein endothelial cells [56]. However, the potentialities of PI-PLC enzymes are far to be completely highlighted.

## PI-PLC Enzymes in Astrocyes

Studies were conducted in order to analyze the role of PI signaling in astrocytes (Table 2). In vitro experiments conducted under different conditions showed that resting (non-activated) rat astrocytes express a selected set of PI-PLC isoforms. That suggested that the enzymes play an important role in the regulation of glial functions [26]. Studies conducted on rat cells demonstrated that PI-PLC isoforms β3, β4, γ1, δ1, δ4, and ε were expressed both in resting neonatal rat astrocytes and in rat astrocytoma C6 cells [26]. Some isoforms were not expressed in astrocytes. Moreover, the expressed isoforms were differently represented in the neoplastic counterpart [26]. This was the case of PI-PLC δ1, which was specifically associated to quiescent astrocytes, while PI-PLC β1 and γ2 isoforms were expressed exclusively by C6 cells. That was substantially in line with the well-known PI-PLC involvement (especially PI-PLC β1) in the progression of the cell cycle [47] and in malignant transformation [26; 35]. In the complex cascade of events involving PI-PLC signaling, the control of cell proliferation seems to be influenced by different expression of isoforms (depending on the cell type), and also by their specific intracellular localization [57]. Immunohistochemical experiments detected marked nuclear localization of PI-PLC β3 isoform both in quiescent and in neoplastic astrocytes, although in C6 it was weakly expressed in the cytoplasm. High specific immunoreactivity of isoforms PI-PLC δ4 and ε in both astrocytes and C6 cells was detected. The expression of PI-PLC δ3 deserves some comment. In fact, PI-PLC δ3, poorly expressed in normal astrocytes [50], was highly expressed in C6 astrocytoma cells, as well as in other neoplastic tissues [49]. That might indicate that up-regulation of PI-PLC δ3 isoform is possible during the neoplastic progression. Further observations corroborated the hypothesis that the different expression of PI-PLC enzymes might be related to neoplastic phenotype progression. In fact, treatment of C6 cells with the specific inhibitor of PI-PLC 1-[6-[[17b-3-methoxyestra-1,3,5(10)-trien-17-yl]amino]exyl]- 1H-pyrrole-2,5-dione (U-73122), an amphiphilic alkylating agent, aminosteroid homologue of the thiol reagent N-ethylmaleimide (NEM), showed interesting results [28]. Treated C6 astrocytoma cells expressed the mRNA of selected isoforms (PI-PLC γ2, PI-PLC δ3, PI-PLC δ4 and PI-PLC ε) 6h after U-73122 treatment, while the remaining isoforms resulted unexpressed. A further study, performed 24h after U-73122 treatment, showed that the PI-PLC expression pattern returned to that observed in untreated C6 cells, excepting for PI-PLC γ2, which remained unexpressed. Therefore, those findings might be related to a transitory decrease/blockade in the transcription of PI-PLC' genes. Likely, the effect of U-73122 lasts less than 24h, although the observations regarding PI-PLC γ2 require further studies [28].

Immunocytochemical analyses were performed in order to describe the distribution of the expressed isoforms within the cell compartments. PI-PLC β1, absent in the nucleus, was detected in the cytoplasm of untreated C6 rat astrocytoma cells 3h after U-73122 administration; after 6h it was no more detected; after 24h it was absent in the nucleus and present in the cytoplasm, resembling the distribution that it had before the U-73122 treatment [28]. PI-PLC β3, present both in the nucleus and in the cytoplasm of untreated C6 rat astrocytoma cells, was not detected after 3 and 6 hours, while it was detected in the cytoplasm 24h after U-73122 treatment [28]. PI-PLC β4, present both in the nucleus and in the cytoplasm of untreated C6 rat astrocytoma cells, was detected in the cytoplasm 3h after U-73122 treatment, and was not detected after 6h; it was detected in the cytoplasm after 24h [28]. PI-PLC γ1 was absent in the nucleus and detected in the cytoplasm of untreated C6 rat astrocytoma cells, and also 3h after U-73122 treatment; it was not detected after 6h; it was absent in the nucleus, and detected in the cytoplasm 24h after U-73122 administration, resembling the distribution that it had before the treatment [28]. PI-PLC γ2, present both in the nucleus and in the cytoplasm of untreated C6 rat astrocytoma cells, was absent in the nucleus and present in the cytoplasm after 3 and 6 hours; it was not detected 24h after U-

73122 treatment. PI-PLC δ3 was present in the nucleus and in the cytoplasm of untreated C6 rat astrocytoma cells, and also after 3 and 6 hours after U-73122 administration; it was absent in the nucleus and present in the cytoplasm 24h after the treatment [28]. PI-PLC δ4 was detected in the nucleus and in the cytoplasm of untreated C6 rat astrocytoma cells, and also 3h after U-73122 administration; it was detected exclusively in the nucleus after 6h, and both in the nucleus and in the cytoplasm 24h after the treatment [28]. PI-PLC ε, present both in the nucleus and in the cytoplasm of untreated C6 rat astrocytoma cells, was present in the nucleus after 3h; it was detected both in the nucleus and in the cytoplasm 6 and 24 hours after U-73122 treatment [28]. The absence of the mRNA of the analyzed isoforms in the period briefly following (3h) the treatment with U-73122 suggests that the inhibiting molecule might interact with the transcription of the genes codifying for the enzymes [28].

Table 2. Expression of pi-plc isoforms in astrocyte cultures in vitro

| Enzymes | astrocytes | LPS treated astrocytes | astrocytoma C6 Cella | U-73122 treated astrocytoma C6 cells |
|---|---|---|---|---|
| PI-PLC β1 | – | + | + | –/+ |
| PI-PLC β2 | – | – | – | – |
| PI-PLC β3 | + | – | + | –/+ |
| PI-PLC β4 | + | + | + | –/+ |
| PI-PLC γ1 | + | + | + | –/+ |
| PI-PLC γ2 | – | – | + | –/+/– |
| PI-PLC δ1 | + | –/+ | – | – |
| PI-PLC δ3 | + | –/+/– | + | –/+ |
| PI-PLC δ4 | + | – | + | –/+ |
| PI-PLC ε | + | – | + | –/+ |

Expression of PI-PLC isoforms (listed in the first column, left) in quiescent neonatal rat astrocytes (second column), activated (LPS treated) neonatal rat astrocytes (third column), rat astrocytoma C6 cells (fourth column), rat astrocytoma C6 cells in which blockade of PI-PLC activity was induced with U-73122 administration.

PI-PLC enzymes were supposed to be involved in the inflammatory activation of astrocytes. Numerous signal transduction pathways were described to be involved in the cascade of events characterizing the inflammation process. Special attention was paid to the production of interleukin 6 (IL-6), involved in the actions induced by endothelin peptides (ETs) [58]. In astrocytes, the ET-G protein mediated PI-PLC activation leads to PI hydrolysis and rapid formation and accumulation of IP3 and DAG [59]. Increase in IL-6 levels was PI-PLC dependent. That did not always require calcium entry, although an agonist of the selective endothelin receptor sub-type B (ETB), named IRL1620, mobilized intracellular calcium content from the cytoplasm stores [60]. Different cytokines and substances like bacterial lipopolysaccharide (LPS) induce the astrocytes to adopt a reactive phenotype. In the presence of LPS, the astrocytes synthesize both IL-6 and TNFα, probably via a PI-PLC dependent pathway. Both the events can be inhibited by LaCl3 and by the PI-PLC agonist U-

73122. In the presence of LPS, addition of the inhibitor showed that the induced cytokine production was PI-PLC dependent and required calcium entry [60]. IRL1620 enhanced the production of IL-6 and TNFα induced by LPS, inducing a significant increase of their levels. Furthermore, IRL1620 also enhanced the LPS induced NO production [60]. The latter effect also required PI-PLC activation [61]. In the presence of LPS, IRL1620 increased nitric oxide synthase (NOS) type II synthesis. The IRL1620 dependent rise of NO production induced by LPS was inhibited by U73122 and LaCl3. That demonstrated that the mechanism used a PI-PLC-dependent activation pathway, depending on calcium entry [60-61].

In recent studies, LPS treatment modified the expression of selected isoforms, such as PI-PLC β3, δ4, and ε. PI-PLC β1, absent in untreated cells, appears after LPS stimulation [27]. PI-PLC δ1 and δ3 were differently expressed after LPS stimulation in a time dependent manner [27]. These observations suggested that PI-PLC enzymes play a role in the modulation (up or down regulation) of astrocytes activation by inflammatory stimulation. In fact, during a 24h observation period after treatment of cultured quiescent astrocytes with LPS, at a very early stage (3h) astrocytes expressed PI-PLC β1 (localized in the nucleus), β4 and γ1 (localized in the cytoplasm) [27]. 6h after LPS stimulation, astrocytes expressed PI-PLC β1, β4 (localized in the cytoplasm), γ1, δ1 (localized both in the nucleus and the cytoplasm), and δ3 (localized in the cytoplasm). 18h after LPS stimulation, astrocytes expressed PI-PLC β1 (localized in the cytoplasm), β4, γ1, and δ1 (localized both in the nucleus and the cytoplasm) [27]. 24h after LPS stimulation, astrocytes expressed PI-PLC β1, δ1, γ1 (localized in the cytoplasm) and β4 (localized both in the nucleus and the cytoplasm). Remarkably, during the period ranging about 6h after LPS treatment, five isoforms (PI-PLC β1, β4, γ1, δ1, and δ3) were contemporarily present within the cytoplasm, two isoforms (PI-PLC γ1 and δ1) were present also within the nucleus [27]. Those observations suggested that the PI-PLC isoforms play a role in the fine tuning in ongoing central nervous system inflammation mimicked by LPS stimulation. PI-PLC might contribute through the temporal modulation of both their expression and sub-cellular distribution [60]. In cells undergone inflammation stimuli, PI-PLC β1, unexpressed in quiescent astrocytes, was expressed; PI-PLC δ3, expressed in quiescent astrocytes, was limitedly expressed (6h after treatment), and PI-PLC β3, δ4, and ε, expressed in quiescent astrocytes, were not expressed. Therefore, the appearing of PI-PLC β1, the brief lasting expression of PI-PLC δ3 and the suppression of PI-PLC β3, δ4, and ε suggested that those isoforms might be involved in the cascade of events leading to astrocyte activation induced by inflammatory stimuli.

## Conclusion

Despite the greatest interest and the considerable research efforts to delineate the metabolic pathways acting in astrocytes, the role of calcium remains to be fully elucidated, as well as the complete panel of molecules involved and the complex regulation mechanisms. Recent evidences indicate that, in astrocytes, the expression panel of PI-PLC isoforms varies under different conditions, such as tumor progression or inflammatory activation, with respect to the quiescent counterpart. These observations suggested that up or down regulation of PI-PLC isoforms contribute to the activation of astrocytes. That also suggests that the PI signal transduction pathway is involved in the activation of the glia and in the ongoing inflammation processes of the nervous system. However, the role of the PI signal transduction pathway in the complex interplay of astrocyes during the neural metabolism requires further studies in order to be elucidated.

# References

[1] Morgan C. J., Pledger W. J. Cell cycle dependent growth factor regulation of gene expression. *J Cell Physiol*. 1989 Dec;141(3):535-42.

[2] Araque A., Parpura V., Sanzgiri R. P., Haydon P. G. Tripartite synapses: glia, the unacknowledged partner. *Trends Neurosci*. 1999 May;22(5):208-15.

[3] Fellin T., Carmignoto G. Neurone-to-astrocyte signalling in the brain represents a distinct multifunctional unit. *J Physiol*. 2004 Aug 15;559(Pt 1):3-15.

[4] Pasti L., Pozzan T., Carmignoto G. Long-lasting changes of calcium oscillations in astrocytes. A new form of glutamate-mediated plasticity. *J Biol Chem*. 1995 Jun 23;270(25):15203-10.

[5] Henneberger C., Papouin T., Oliet S. H., Rusakov D. A. Long-term potentiation depends on release of D-serine from astrocytes. *Nature*. 2010 Jan 14;463(7278):232-6.

[6] Perea G, Araque A. Glial calcium signaling and neuron-glia communication. *Cell Calcium*. 2005 Sep-Oct;38(3-4):375-82.

[7] Serrano A., Haddjeri N., Lacaille J. C., Robitaille R. GABAergic network activation of glial cells underlies hippocampal heterosynaptic depression. *J Neurosci*. 2006 May 17;26(20):5370-82.

[8] Halassa M. M., Haydon P. G. Integrated brain circuits: astrocytic networks modulate neuronal activity and behavior. *Annu Rev Physiol*. 2010 Mar 17;72:335-55.

[9] Volterra A., Meldolesi J. Astrocytes, from brain glue to communication elements: the revolution continues. *Nat Rev Neurosci*. 2005 Aug;6(8):626-40.

[10] D'Ascenzo M., Podda M. V., Fellin T., Azzena G. B., Haydon P., Grassi C. Activation of mGluR5 induces spike afterdepolarization and enhanced excitability in medium spiny neurons of the nucleus accumbens by modulating persistent $Na^+$ currents. *J Physiol*. 2009 Jul 1;587(Pt 13):3233-50.

[11] Honsek S. D., Walz C., Kafitz K. W., Rose C. R. Astrocyte calcium signals at Schaffer collateral to CA1 pyramidal cell synapses correlate with the number of activated synapses but not with synaptic strength. *Hippocampus*. 2010 Sep 29. doi: 10.1002/hipo.20843.

[12] Grosche J, Matyash V, Möller T, Verkhratsky A, Reichenbach A, Kettenmann H. Microdomains for neuron-glia interaction: parallel fiber signaling to Bergmann glial cells. *Nat Neurosci*. 1999 Feb;2(2):139-43.

[13] Bergles D. E., Jahr C. E. Synaptic activation of glutamate transporters in hippocampal astrocytes. *Neuron*. 1997 Dec;19(6):1297-308.

[14] Todd K. J., Darabid H., Robitaille R. Perisynaptic glia discriminate patterns of motor nerve activity and influence plasticity at the neuromuscular junction. *J Neurosci*. 2010 Sep 1;30(35):11870-82.

[15] Fox P. T., Raichle M. E., Mintun M. A., Dence C. Nonoxidative glucose consumption during focal physiologic neural activity. *Science*. 1988 Jul 22;241(4864):462-4.

[16] Fox P. T., Raichle M. E. Focal physiological uncoupling of cerebral blood flow and oxidative metabolism during somatosensory stimulation in human subjects. *Proc Natl Acad Sci U S A*. 1986 Feb;83(4):1140-4.

[17] Barinaga M. New imaging methods provide a better view into the brain. *Science*. 1997 Jun 27;276(5321):1974-6.

[18] Prichard J., Rothman D., Novotny E., Petroff O., Kuwabara T., Avison M., Howseman A., Hanstock C., Shulman R. Lactate rise detected by 1H NMR in human visual cortex during physiologic stimulation. *Proc Natl Acad Sci USA*. 1991 Jul 1;88(13):5829-31.

[19] Walz W., Mukerji S. Lactate release from cultured astrocytes and neurons: a comparison. *Glia*. 1988;1(6):366-70.

[20] Pellerin L., Magistretti P. J. Glutamate uptake into astrocytes stimulates aerobic glycolysis: a mechanism coupling neuronal activity to glucose utilization. Proc Natl Acad Sci U S A. 1994 Oct 25;91(22):10625-9.

[21] Raichle M. E., Gusnard D. A. Appraising the brain's energy budget. *Proc Natl Acad Sci U S A*. 2002 Aug 6;99(16):10237-9.

[22] Schwartz I. R., Bok D. Electron microscopic localization of [125I]alpha-bungarotoxin binding sites in the outer plexiform layer of the goldfish retina. *J Neurocytol*. 1979 Feb;8(1):53-66.

[23] Roy C. S., Sherrington C. S. On the Regulation of the Blood-supply of the Brain. *J Physiol*. 1890 Jan;11(1-2):85-158.17.

[24] Schummers J., Yu H., Sur M. Tuned responses of astrocytes and their influence on hemodynamic signals in the visual cortex. *Science*. 2008 Jun 20;320(5883):1638-43.

[25] Carmignoto G., Gómez-Gonzalo M. The contribution of astrocyte signalling to neurovascular coupling. *Brain Res Rev*. 2010 May;63(1-2):138-48.

[26] Lo Vasco V. R., Fabrizi C., Artico M., Cocco L., Billi A. M., Fumagalli L, Manzoli FA. Expression of phosphoinositide-specific phospholipase C isoenzymes in cultured astrocytes. *J Cell Biochem*, 2007, 100(4), 952-959.

[27] Lo Vasco V. R., Fabrizi C., Fumagalli L., Cocco L. Expression of phosphoinositide specific phospholipase C isoenzymes in cultured astrocytes activated after stimulation with Lipopolysaccharide. *J Cell Biochem*, 2010, 109(5), 1006-1012.

[28] Lo Vasco V. R., Fabrizi C., Panetta B., Fumagalli L., Cocco L. Expression pattern and sub cellular distribution of Phosphoinositide specific Phospholipase C enzymes after treatment with U-73122 in rat astrocytoma cells. *J Cell Biochem*, 2010 110(4):1005-1012.

[29] Hokin M. R., Hokin L. E. Enzyme secretion and the incorporation of P32 into phospholipides of pancreas slices. *J Biol Chem*. 1953 Aug;203(2):967-77.

[30] Sekar M. C., Hokin L. E. **Phosphoinositide metabolism and cGMP levels are not coupled to the muscarinic-cholinergic receptor in human erythrocyte.** *Life Sci*. 1986 Oct 6;39(14):1257-62.

[31] Irvine R. F. 2002. Nuclear lipid signalling. *Sci STKE* 150:RE13.

[32] Noh D. Y., Shin S. H., Rhee S. G. Phosphoinositide-specific phospholipase C and mitogenic signalling. *Biochim Biophys Acta*. 1995. 1242: 99-114.

[33] Suh P. G., Park J., Manzoli L., Cocco L., Peak J. C., Katan M., Fukami K., Kataoka T., Yuk S., Ryu S. H. 2008. Multiple roles of phosphoinositide-specific phospholipase C isozymes. *BMB Reports* 41:415-434.

[34] Cocco L., Faenza I., Follo M. Y., Billi A. M., Ramazzotti G., Papa V., Martelli A. M., Manzoli L. Nuclear inositides: PI-PLC signaling in cell growth, differentiation and pathology. *Adv Enzyme Regul.* 2009, 49(1):2-10.

[35] Lo Vasco V. R., Calabrese G., Manzoli L., Palka G., Spadano A., Morizio E., Guanciali-Franchi P., Fantasia D., Cocco L. Inositide-specific phospholipase c beta1 gene deletion in the progression of myelodysplastic syndrome to acute myeloid leukemia. *Leukemia.* 2004, 18(6):1122-6.

[36] Pandey G. N., Dwivedi Y., Pandey S. C., Teas S. S., Conley R. R., Roberts R. C., Tamminga C. A. Low phosphoinositide-specific phospholipase C activity and expression of phospholipase C beta1 protein in the prefrontal cortex of teenage suicide subjects. *Am J Psychiatry.* 1999, 156(12):1895–1901.

[37] Rípová D., Strunecká A., Nemcová V., Farská I. Phospholipids and calcium alterations in platelets of schizophrenic patients. *Physiol Res.* 1997, 46(1):59–68.

[38] Lin X. H., Kitamura N., Hashimoto T., Shirakawa O., Maeda K. Opposite changes in phosphoinositide-specific phospholipase C immunoreactivity in the left prefrontal and superior temporal cortex of patients with chronic schizophrenia. *Biol Psychiatry.* 1999, 46 (12):1665–1671.

[39] Lo Vasco V. R., Cardinale G., Polonia P. Deletion of PLCB1 gene in schizophrenia affected patients. *J Cell Mol Med* epub 2011 22th June. doi: 10.1111/j.1469-445X.2011.01363.x.

[40] Udawela M., Scarr E., Hannan A. J., Thomas E. A., Dean B. Phospholipase C beta 1 expression in the dorsolateral prefrontal cortex from patients with schizophrenia at different stages of illness. *Aust N Z J Psychiatry.* 2011 Feb;45(2):140-7.

[41] Nakamura Y., Fukami K. Roles of phospholipase C isozymes in organogenesis and embryonic development. *Physiology* (2009) 24:332–341.

[42] Comer F. I., Parent C. A. Phosphoinositides specify polarity during epithelial organ development. *Cell* (2007) 128(2):239–240.

[43] Hisatsune C., Nakamura K., Kuroda Y, Nakamura T, Mikoshiba K. Amplification of $Ca^{2+}$ signaling by diacylglycerol-mediated inositol 1,4,5-trisphosphate production. *J Biol Chem* 2005. 280(12):11723-30.

[44] Bunney T. D., Katan M. PLC regulation: emerging pictures for molecular mechanisms. *Trends Biochem Sci.* 2011 Feb;36(2):88-96.

[45] Tanaka O., Kondo H. 1994. Localization of mRNAs for three novel members (beta 3, beta 4 and gamma 2) of phospholipase C family in mature rat brain. *Neurosci Lett* 182:17–20.

[46] Adamski F. M., Timms K. M., Shieh B. H. 1999. A unique isoform of phospholipase Cbeta4 highly expressed in the cerebellum and eye. *Biochim Biophys Acta* 1444:55–60.

[47] Yamaga M., Fujii M., Kamata H., Hirata H., Yagisawa H. 1999. Phospholipase C-delta1 contains a functional nuclear export signal sequence. *J Biol Chem* 274:28537–28541.

[48] Mao G. F., Kunapuli S. P., Koneti Rao A. 2000. Evidence for two alternatively spliced forms of phospholipase C-beta2 in haematopoietic cells. *Br J Haematol* 110:402–408.

[49] Pawelczyk T., Matecki A. 1998. Localization of phospholipase C delta3 in the cell and regulation of its activity by phospholipids and calcium. *Eur J Biochem* 257:169–177.

[50] Pawelczyk T. 1999. Isozymes delta of phosphoinositidespecific phospholipase C. *Acta Biochim Pol* 46:91–98.

[51] Ananthanarayanan B., Das S., Rhee S. G., Murray D., Cho W. 2002. Membrane targeting of C2 domains of phospholipase C-delta isoforms. *J Biol Chem* 277:3568–3575.

[52] McBride K., Rhee S. G., Jaken S. 1991. Immunocytochemical localization of phospholipase C-gamma in rat embryo fibroblasts. *Proc Natl Acad Sci USA* 88(16):7111-5.

[53] Diakonova M., Chilov D., Arnaoutov A., Alexeyev V., Nikolsky N., Medvedeva N. 1997. Intracellular distribution of phospholipase C gamma 1 in cell lines with different levels of transformation. *Eur J Cell Biol* 73:360–367.

[54] Wing M. R., Bourdon D. M., Harden T. K. 2003. PLC-epsilon: a shared effector protein in Ras-, Rho-, and G alpha beta gamma-mediated signaling. *Mol Interv* 3:273–280.

[55] Saunders C. M., Larman M. G., Parrington J., Cox L. J., Royse J., Blayney L. M., Swann K., Lai F. A. 2002. PLC zeta: a sperm-specific trigger of Ca(2+) oscillations in egs and embryo development. *Development* 129:3533-3544.

[56] Lo Vasco V. R., Pacini L., Di Raimo T., D'Arcangelo D., Businaro R. Expression of Phosphoinositide-specific phospholipase C isoforms in HUVEC. *J Clin Pathol*. Epub 8 July 2011.

[57] Santi P., Solimando L., Zini N., Santi S., Riccio M., Guidotti L. 2003. Inositol-specific phospholipase C in low and fast proliferating hepatoma cell lines. *Int J Oncol* 22:1147–1153.

[58] Rubanyi G.M., Polokoff M.A. 1994. Endothelins: molecular biology, biochemistry, pharmacology, physiology and pathophysiology. *Pharmacol Rev*; 46(3): 325-415.

[59] MacCumber M.W., Ross C.A., Snyder S.H. 1990. Endothelin in brain: receptors, mitogenesis and biosynthesis in glial cells. *Proc Natl Acad Sci* USA; 87(6):2359-63.

[60] Morga E., Faber C., Heuschling P. 2000. Stimulation of Endothelin B Receptor modulates the inflammatory activation of rat astrocytes. *J Neurochem* 603-612.

[61] Wang H., Reiser G. 2003. Signal transduction by serine proteinases in astrocytes: regulation of proliferation, morphologic changes, and survival via proteinase-activated receptors. *Drug Devel Res* 60:43-50.

In: Astrocytes
Editor: Oscar González-Pérez

ISBN: 978-1-62081-558-8
© 2012 Nova Science Publishers, Inc.

*Chapter IV*

# Astrocytes as Neural Stem Cells in the Adult Brain

### Oscar Gonzalez-Perez[*]
Laboratory of Neuroscience, Facultad de Psicologia,
Universidad de Colima, Colima, Mexico
Department of Neuroscience, Centro Universitario de Ciencias
de la Salud, Universidad de Guadalajara. Guadalajara, Jal, México

## Abstract

In the adult mammalian brain, *bona fide* neural stem cells were discovered in the subventricular zone (SVZ), the largest neurogenic niche lining the striatal wall of the lateral ventricles of the brain. In this region resides a subpopulation of astrocytes that express the glial fibrillary acidic protein (GFAP), nestin and carbohydrate Lewis X (LeX). Astonishingly, these GFAP-expressing progenitors display stem-cell-like features both *in vivo* and *in vitro*. Throughout life SVZ astrocytes give rise to interneurons and oligodendrocyte precursors, which populate the olfactory bulb and the white matter, respectively. The role of the progenies of SVZ astrocytes has not been fully elucidated, but some evidence indicates that the new neurons play a role in olfactory discrimination, whereas oligodendrocytes contribute to myelinate white matter tracts. In this chapter, we describe the astrocytic nature of adult neural stem cells, their organization into the SVZ and some of their molecular and genetic characteristics.

## Introduction

In 1931, Santiago Ramon y Cajal stated "The Nature has granted us with a limited endowment of cerebral cells. This is a resource, large or little, which nobody can increase because the neuron is unable to reproduce itself" (Cajal's speech for the *Archivo de la*

---

[*] Oscar Gonzalez-Perez, M.D., Ph.D.; Facultad de Psicologia Universidad de Colima; Av. Universidad # 333; Colima, COL 28040; Mexico; E-mail: osglez@gmail.com and/or osglez@ucol.mx.

*Palabra*, Spain). This statement soon became a dogma that was passionately supported by many other prominent neuroscientists. However, at the 1960's, Joseph Altman (Altman, 1962) challenged this assumption by showing that the postnatal brain was not a quiescent organ incapable of neurogenesis. In a series of experiments Altman and colleagues, as well as other groups, described the presence of neurons labeled with tritiated thymidine (*3H-TdR*) in the subependymal zone lining the lateral wall of the lateral ventricles, which suggested the presence of neurogenesis in the adult brain (Altman and Gopal, 1965; Altman and Das, 1967; Kaplan and Hinds, 1977). Later studies from other groups also described ongoing neurogenesis in female canaries (Goldman and Nottebohm, 1983) and lizards (Pérez-Cañellas and García-Verdugo, 1996). Since 3H-TdR may also induce cell cycle arrest and apoptosis, these initial results were somehow criticized and could not unequivocally determine the presence of neurogenesis in the adult brain. This controversy was finally finished by Arturo Alvarez-Buylla and coworkers, whom in serial experiments not only demonstrated the presence of new born neurons (neuroblasts) *in vivo*, but also proved that the primary progenitor of these neuroblasts is a subpopulation of astrocytes resident in the lateral walls of the lateral ventricles of the adult mammalian brain. These newly generated cells migrate anteriorly and form functional circuits with the resident neurons in the olfactory bulb (Lois and Alvarez-Buylla, 1993, 1994a; Lois et al., 1996; Doetsch et al., 1997; Wichterle et al., 1997; Doetsch et al., 1999b; Sanai et al., 2004; Spassky et al., 2005; Jackson et al., 2006; Merkle et al., 2007).

Since the discovery of neurogenesis in the adult mammalian brain, a lot of research has been done in several brain regions to determine the presence new born neurons but, so far, it is well-accepted that this process is mainly confined to the subventricular zone (*SVZ*) at the forebrain and the subgranular zone (*SGZ*) in the dentate gyrus at the hippocampus (Reznikov, 1991; Luskin, 1993; Lois and Alvarez-Buylla, 1994b). The SVZ is the largest neurogenic niche in the adult mammalian brain (Luskin, 1993; Alvarez-Buylla and Garcia-Verdugo, 2002). In this region resides a subpopulation of glial cells with stem-cell-like features, both *in vivo* and *in vitro*, which can give rise to neurons, oligodendrocytes, NG2-glia and astrocytes (Doetsch et al., 1999c; Laywell et al., 2000; Imura et al., 2003; Morshead et al., 2003; Garcia et al., 2004; Menn et al., 2006; Gonzalez-Perez et al., 2009; Gonzalez-Perez and Quinones-Hinojosa, 2010; Gonzalez-Perez and Alvarez-Buylla, 2011). The role of the new born neurons and oligodendrocytes derived from the adult SVZ has not been fully elucidated, but some evidence indicates that the new neurons play a role in odor discrimination tasks (Gheusi et al., 2000), whereas SVZ oligodendrocyte precursors contribute to maintain the population of oligodendrocytes in the white matter (Menn et al., 2006; Gonzalez-Perez et al., 2009; Gonzalez-Perez and Alvarez-Buylla, 2011).

In contrast to the SVZ progenitors, the precursor cells found in the SGZ of dentate gyrus in the hippocampus appear not to be *bona fide* neural stem cells, because they only give rise to neurons *in vivo*. In fact, some studies showed that adult SGZ progenitors were not multipotent self-renewing progenitors (Seaberg and van der Kooy, 2002; Bull and Bartlett, 2005). Therefore, SGZ neurogenic progenitors are not considered neural stem cells, but neuronal precursor cells (Song et al., 2002; Jagasia et al., 2006). In this chapter, I discuss the characteristics and functions of adult neural stem cells *per se*, as well as, I describe the evidence that demonstrated the astrocytic identity of multipotent cells resident within the adult SVZ.

# Neural Stem Cells in the Adult Brain

Early experiments *in vitro* found that tissue harvested from the SVZ contained a subpopulation of multipotent precursor cells, which under growth-factor-enriched conditions were able to produce self-renewing clones (Reynolds and Weiss, 1992; Morshead et al., 1994; Weiss et al., 1996). These clones proliferated and gave rise to spherical cell aggregates known as '*neurospheres*', which if subsequently subjected to growth factor removal and serum-free conditions, formed neurons, oligodendrocytes, and astrocytes, suggesting that these self-renewing cells are also multipotent. In consequence, the neurosphere assay has been extensively utilized as a method to indicate the presence of stem cells in tissue samples. However, more recent evidence indicates that this assay might not accurately identify stem cell capacity *in vivo*. Therefore *in vivo* experiments are always required to fully demonstrate the '*stemness*' potential in the mammalian brain. The capacity of SVZ progenitor cells to behave as putative stem cells *in vivo* was subsequently demonstrated in rodents and humans (Doetsch et al., 1999b; Laywell et al., 2000; Sanai et al., 2004).

The presence of *bona fide* neural stem cells in the adult brain has been demonstrated through multiple experimental approaches. Primary precursors were identified *in vivo* by using deoxythymidine or bromodeoxyuridine (*BrdU*) as cell proliferation markers. Thus, it was found that a subpopulation of astrocytes remain labeled into the SVZ and SGZ after long survival times, which suggested that these glial cells corresponded to stem cells (Doetsch et al., 1999b; Alvarez-Buylla et al, 2002). These multipotent astrocytes are denominated as *type-B cells*, which typically express the glial fibrillary acidic protein (*GFAP*) and have very well-defined ultrastructural characteristics (see Chapter 5). The first evidence indicating that SVZ astrocytes are neural stem cells was provided by Fiona Doetsch et al. They discovered that a subpopulation of astrocytes that survived to an intracerebroventricular administration of a cytotoxic drug (cytosine-β-D-arabinofuranoside, *Ara-C*) was able to fully regenerate all germinal progenitors within the SVZ over a period of 14 days (Doetsch et al, 1999b; Doetsch et al, 1999a). After that, also using Ara-C to identify the primary progenitor in the SGZ, Betina Seri et al. found that SGZ radial astrocytes (named *type-D* cells) were capable of reconstituting the germinal layers in the dentate gyrus (Seri et al., 2001). Later reports confirmed these observations indicating that the GFAP-expressing astrocytes are candidate stem cells in the SVZ (Chiasson et al, 1999; Capela and Temple, 2002; Garcia et al, 2004; Spassky et al, 2005). Interestingly, astrocytes collected from multiple brain regions before postnatal day 10 may behave as neural stem cells *in vitro*. After that time, only the SVZ astrocytes retain this '*stemness*' capacity (Lim and Alvarez-Buylla, 1999; Laywell et al., 2000).

# Organization of the Subventricular Zone

The subventricular zone, the largest niche of adult neural stem cells, is located along the lateral walls of the lateral ventricles in the forebrain (Figure 1) (Doetsch et al., 1997; Doetsch, 2003). To have a complete view of the SVZ as a neurogenic niche, we have to study not only the cell organization and ultrastructure of the SVZ progenitors, but also their interrelationships with surrounding microenvironment. Thus, some authors have denominated the SVZ niche as the ventricular-subventicular (VZ-SVZ) compartment (Mirzadeh et al., 2008). For the purposes of this chapter we will refer to this region simply as the SVZ. The adult SVZ has a center-surround cell arrangement, denominated as 'pinwheel' organization, for ependymal cells (type-E cells) and astrocytes (type-B cells) within ventricular walls (Mirzadeh et al., 2008). These pinwheel-like compartments contain the apical endings of type-B cells and of multiciliated (type-E1) and bi-ciliated (type-E2) ependymal cells (Figure 1). Remarkably, SVZ astrocytes extend two cell processes: a petite cilium that contact the ventricular lumen and a long basal process attached to blood vessels (Figure 1)(Mirzadeh et al., 2008; Shen et al., 2008). Some authors have proposed that these contacts are important to regulate adult neurogenesis through signals derived from extracellular matrix proteins, soluble factors or blood-vessel secretion (Leventhal et al., 1999; Mercier et al., 2002; Shen et al., 2008; Tavazoie et al., 2008). Some of these chemical mediators include the CXC chemokine, the stromal-derived factor 1 (*SDF-1*), the epidermal (*EGF*), the platelet-derived (*PDGF*) and the fibroblast (*FGF*) growth factors (Reynolds and Weiss, 1992; Vescovi et al., 1993; Gritti et al., 1995; Craig et al., 1996; Gritti et al., 1999; Jackson et al., 2006; Kokovay et al., 2010).

Interestingly, the cell organization of the adult human SVZ is quite different to that found in rodents and most of the mammalians. In the human SVZ, astrocytes are not adjacent to the ependymal, instead, they accumulate into the parenchyma and form a 'ribbon' of cells separated from the ependymal layer by a gap that is largely devoid of cell bodies (Sanai et al., 2004; Quinones-Hinojosa et al., 2006).

## SVZ Astrocytes as Neural Stem Cells

The adult SVZ contains slowly dividing type-B cells, the putative neural stem cells, which are a subpopulation of astrocytes that expresses nestin, GFAP and carbohydrate Lewis X (*LeX*) (Doetsch et al., 1999b; Rietze et al., 2001; Capela and Temple, 2002; Garcia et al., 2004). Type-B astrocytes divide to self-renew and generate highly proliferating transit-amplifying progenitors (type-C cells), which in turn produce neuroblasts (type-A cells) (Figure 1 and 2) (Doetsch et al., 1997; Doetsch et al., 1999b). The cytoplasmic processes of type B cells sheath type-A cells and contribute to form tangential neuroblast chains. The confluence of neuroblast chains forms a brain structure, called the rostral migratory stream *(RMS)*, which goes through the olfactory tract and connects the anterior SVZ with the olfactory bulb (Figure 2) (Lois and Alvarez-Buylla, 1994a; Lois et al., 1996). Once in the olfactory bulb, type-A cells differentiate into mature neuronal cells that continually replace interneurons in the glomerular and the mitral cell layers (Lois and Alvarez-Buylla, 1993, 1994a; Merkle et al., 2007).

Remarkably, type-B stem cells are not a homogeneous population; instead, it seems they comprise restricted subpopulations with diverse neurogenic potential (Merkle et al., 2007). In addition to interneurons, type-B astrocytes of the SVZ produce oligodendrocyte precursor cells that help maintain the oligodendrocyte population in the corpus callosum, fimbria fornix and striatum (Menn et al., 2006; Gonzalez-Perez et al., 2009; Gonzalez-Perez and Quinones-Hinojosa, 2010; Gonzalez-Perez and Alvarez-Buylla, 2011)

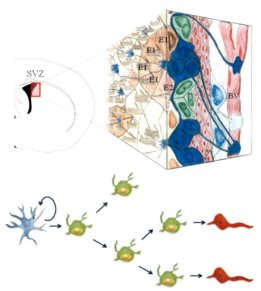

Reprinted from Brain Research Reviews, Vol 67, Gonzalez-Perez & Alvarez-Buylla, Oligodendrogenesis in the subventricular zone and the role of epidermal growth factor, page 148, Copyright 2011, with permission from Elsevier.

Figure 1. The adult subventricular zone (SVZ) is lining the striatal wall of the lateral ventricles in the brain (coronal section left). A 3-D model of the SVZ is shown to the right. This region contains astrocytic neural stem cells (type-B cells depicted in blue). Type-B cells give rise to rapidly dividing intermediate progenitor cells (type-C cells depicted in green), which in turn produce migrating neuroblasts (type-A cells depicted in red). Type-B astrocytes have a long basal process contacting blood vessels (BV) and an apical ending at the ventricle surface. Note the pinwheel-like organization composed of multiciliated (Type-E1) and bi-ciliated (Type-E2) ependymal cells encircling apical surfaces of astrocytes.

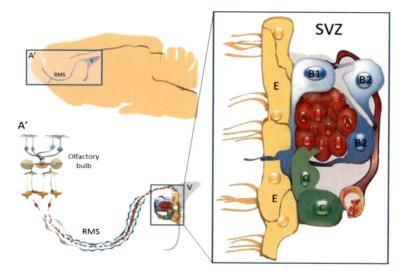

Figure 2. Cellular organization of the adult subventricular zone (SVZ), rostral migratory stream (RMS) and the olfactory bulb. Neuroblast (type-A cells) in the SVZ migrate to the olfactory bulb via the RMS. Migrating neuroblasts differentiate into granular and periglomerular interneurons in the olfactory bulb. B1: Type-B1 cell; B2: parenchymal astrocyte; C: Type-C cell; A: Type-A cell; E: Ependymal cells; V: Ventricle.

The identification of type-B cells in the SVZ as primary neural progenitors of new neurons and oligodendrocytes was demonstrated by labeling SVZ astrocytes in transgenic mice denominated as GFAP-tva mice (Figure 3) (Doetsch et al., 1999b; Doetsch et al., 2002; Menn et al., 2006). These animals express the receptor for an avian leukosis retrovirus (RCAS) controlled by the GFAP gene promoter (Holland and Varmus, 1998). Thus, the progeny of dividing astrocytes can be permanently traced by injecting engineered avian RCAS retroviruses carrying an inheritable reporter gene, which drives the expression of green fluorescent protein. With this method, it has been demonstrated that type-B astrocytes *in vivo* can generate both new neurons and new oligodendrocytes, and both of them become permanent and functional populations of cells in the adult brain (Doetsch et al., 1999b; Menn et al., 2006; Gonzalez-Perez et al., 2009). Interestingly, parenchymal astrocytes from cortex, striatum, septum or white matter appear not to have multipotential properties.

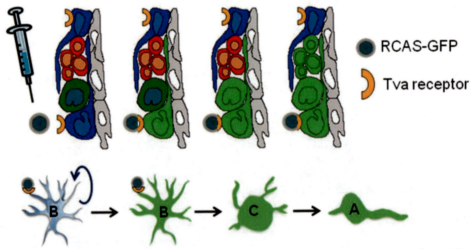

Reprinted from Brain Research Reviews, Vol 67, Gonzalez-Perez & Alvarez-Buylla, Oligodendrogenesis in the subventricular zone and the role of epidermal growth factor, page 150, Copyright 2011, with permission from Elsevier.

Figure 3. Schematic representation of the RCAS/GFAP-tva system. After injection of the RCAS-GFP virus, proliferating astrocytes incorporate into their genome the gene of green fluorescent protein, which is inherited to their progeny. With this system only dividing GFAP-expressing cells are permanently label and can be efficiently traced throughout life.

After these initial reports, other studies using viral transfection or mutant mice have fully demonstrated that GFAP-expressing astrocytes are neural stem cells in the adult mammalian brain. Conditional ablation of GFAP-expressing cells produces a complete loss of neurogenesis (Imura et al., 2003; Morshead et al., 2003). Interestingly, a recent study using a Cre-lox-based strategy demonstrated that radial glial cells (multipotent neural precursors in the developing brain) and SVZ zone astrocytes (multipotent neural precursors in the adult brain) belong to the same lineage (Merkle et al., 2004). This study showed that radial glial cells generate SVZ astrocytes, which act as adult neural stem cells both *in vivo* and *in vitro*. Taken together, these findings confirm that SVZ astrocytes function as neural stem cells in the adult brain.

## Conclusion

A subpopulation of astrocytes derived from the SVZ acts as neural stem cells both *in vivo* and *in vitro*. These findings have changed our perception about glia and though we have greatly advanced our understanding of neural stem cells, there are still many unanswered questions. For instance, what are the fundamental characteristics that distinguish neurogenic astrocytes from the vast population of non-neurogenic astrocytes elsewhere in the brain? What genetic profiles induce SVZ astrocytes to act as a stem cell? Can SVZ astrocytes be induced to generate a specific repertoire of neural cell types? Addressing these questions may shed light on the genetic and molecular basis of stem-cell behavior in SVZ astrocytes, which in turn will allow designing novel therapies against neurodegenerative diseases.

## Acknowledgments

This work was supported by grants from the Consejo Nacional de Ciencia y Tecnologia (CONACyT; CB-2008-101476) and The National Institute of Health and the National Institute of Neurological Disorders and Stroke (NIH/NINDS; R01 NS070024). I also thank to Jimena Rocha-Espejel for her technical assistance.

## References

Altman J. (1962) Are new neurons formed in the brains of adult mammals? *Science* 135:1127-1128.

Altman J., Gopal DD (1965) Post-natal origin of microneurones in the rat brain. *Nature* 207:953-956.

Altman J., Das G. D. (1967) Autoradiographic and Histological Studies of Postnatal Neurogenesis. I. A Longitudinal Investigation of the Kinetics, Migration and Transformation of Cells Incorporating Tritiated Thymidine in Neonate Rats, with Special Reference to Postnatal Neurogenesis in Some Brain Regions. *J CompNeurol* 126:337-390.

Alvarez-Buylla A., Garcia-Verdugo J. M. (2002) Neurogenesis in adult subventricular zone. *J Neurosci* 22:629-634.

Alvarez-Buylla A., Seri B, Doetsch F (2002) Identification of neural stem cells in the adult vertebrate brain. *Brain Res Bull* 57:751-758.

Bull N. D, Bartlett P. F. (2005) The adult mouse hippocampal progenitor is neurogenic but not a stem cell. *J Neurosci* 25:10815-10821.

Capela A., Temple S. (2002) LeX/ssea-1 is expressed by adult mouse CNS stem cells, identifying them as nonependymal. *Neuron* 35:865-875.

Craig C. G., Tropepe V., Morshead C. M., Reynolds B. A., Weiss S., Van der Kooy D. (1996) *In vivo* growth factor expansion of endogenous subependymal neural precursor cell populations in the adult mouse brain. *J Neurosci* 16:2649-2658.

Chiasson B. J., Tropepe V., Morshead C. M., Van der Kooy D. (1999) Adult Mammalian Forebrain Ependymal and Subependymal Cells Demonstrate Proliferative Potential, but only Subependymal Cells Have Neural Stem Cell Characteristics. *J Neurosci* 19:4462-4471.

Doetsch F. (2003) The glial identity of neural stem cells. *Nat Neurosci* 6:1127-1134.

Doetsch F., Garcia-Verdugo J. M., Alvarez-Buylla A. (1997) Cellular composition and three-dimensional organization of the subventricular germinal zone in the adult mammalian brain. *J Neurosci* 17:5046-5061.

Doetsch F., Garcia-Verdugo J. M., Alvarez-Buylla A. (1999a) Regeneration of a germinal layer in the adult mammalian brain. *Proc Nat lAcad Sci USA* 96:11619-11624.

Doetsch F., Caille I., Lim D. A., García-Verdugo J. M., Alvarez-Buylla A. (1999b) Subventricular Zone Astrocytes Are Neural Stem Cells in the Adult mammalian Brain. *Cell* 97:1-20.

Doetsch F., Caille I., Lim D. A., Garcia-Verdugo J. M., Alvarez-Buylla A. (1999c) Subventricular zone astrocytes are neural stem cells in the adult mammalian brain. *Cell* 97:703-716.

Doetsch F., Petreanu L., Caille I., Garcia-Verdugo J. M., Alvarez-Buylla A. (2002) EGF converts transit-amplifying neurogenic precursors in the adult brain into multipotent stem cells. *Neuron* 36:1021-1034.

Garcia A. D., Doan N. B., Imura T., Bush T. G., Sofroniew M. V. (2004) GFAP-expressing progenitors are the principal source of constitutive neurogenesis in adult mouse forebrain. *Nat Neurosci* 7:1233-1241.

Gheusi G., Cremer H., McLean H., Chazal G., Vincent J. D., Lledo P. M (2000) Importance of newly generated neurons in the adult olfactory bulb for odor discrimination. *Proc Natl Acad Sci USA* 97:1823-1828.

Goldman S. A., Nottebohm F. (1983) Neuronal production, migration, and differentiation in a vocal control nucleus of the adult female canary brain. *Proc Natl Acad Sci USA* 80:2390-2394.

Gonzalez-Perez O., Quinones-Hinojosa A. (2010) Dose-dependent effect of EGF on migration and differentiation of adult subventricular zone astrocytes. *Glia* 58:975-983.

Gonzalez-Perez O., Alvarez-Buylla A. (2011) Oligodendrogenesis in the subventricular zone and the role of epidermal growth factor. *Brain Res Rev* 67:147-156.

Gonzalez-Perez O., Romero-Rodriguez R., Soriano-Navarro M., Garcia-Verdugo J. M., Alvarez-Buylla A. (2009) Epidermal Growth Factor Induces the Progeny of Subventricular Zone Type B Cells to Migrate and Differentiate into Oligodendrocytes. *Stem Cells* 27:2032-2043.

Gritti A., Cova L., Parati E. A., Galli R., Vescovi A. L. (1995) Basic fibroblast growth factor supports the proliferation of epidermal growth factor-generated neuronal precursor cells of the adult mouse CNS. *NeurosciLett* 185:151-154.

Gritti A., Frolichsthal-Schoeller P., Galli R, Parati E. A., Cova L., Pagano S. F., Bjornson C. R. R., Vescovi A. L. (1999) Epidermal and fibroblast growth factors behave as mitogenic regulators for a single multipotent stem cell-like population from the subventricular region of the adult mouse forebrain. *J Neurosci* 19:3287-3297.

Holland E. C., Varmus H. E. (1998) Basic fibroblast growth factor induces cell migration and proliferation after glia-specific gene transfer in mice. *Proc Natl Acad Sci USA* 95:1218-1223.

Imura T., Kornblum H I., Sofroniew M. V. (2003) The Predominant Neural Stem Cell Isolated from Postnatal and Adult Forebrain But Not Early Embryonic Forebrain Expresses GFAP. *J Neurosci* 23:2824-2832.

Jackson E. L., Garcia-Verdugo J. M., Gil-Perotin S., Roy M., Quinones-Hinojosa A., VandenBerg S., Alvarez-Buylla A. (2006) PDGFR alpha-positive B cells are neural stem cells in the adult SVZ that form glioma-like growths in response to increased PDGF signaling. *Neuron* 51:187-199.

Jagasia R., Song H., Gage F. H., Lie D. C. (2006) New regulators in adult neurogenesis and their potential role for repair. *Trends Mol Med* 12:400-405.

Kaplan M. S., Hinds J. W. (1977) Neurogenesis in the adult rat: Electron microscopic analysis of light radioautographs. *Science* 197:1092-1094.

Kokovay E., Goderie S., Wang Y., Lotz S., Lin G., Sun Y., Roysam B., Shen Q., Temple S. (2010) Adult S. V. Z. Lineage cells home to and leave the vascular niche via differential responses to SDF1/CXCR4 signaling. *Cell Stem Cell* 7:163-173.

Laywell E. D., Rakic P., Kukekov V. G., Holland E. C., Steindler D. A. (2000) Identification of a multipotent astrocytic stem cell in the immature and adult mouse brain. *Proc Natl Acad Sci USA* 97:13883-13888.

Leventhal C., Rafii S., Rafii D., Shahar A., Goldman S. (1999) Endothelial Trophic Support of Neuronal Production and Recruitment from the Adult Mammalian Subependyma. *Mol Cell Neurosci* 13:450-464.

Lim D. A., Alvarez-Buylla A. (1999) Interaction between astrocytes and adult subventricular zone precursors stimulates neurogenesis. *Proc Natl Acad Sci USA* 96. 96:7526-7531.

Lois C., Alvarez-Buylla A. (1993) Proliferating subventricular zone cells in the adult mammalian forebrain can differentiate into neurons and glia. *Proc Natl Acad Sci USA* 90:2074-2077.

Lois C., Alvarez-Buylla A. (1994a) Long-distance neuronal migration in the adult mammalian brain. *Science* 264:1145-1148.

Lois C., Alvarez-Buylla A. (1994b) Long-distance neuronal migration in the adult mammalian brain. *Science* 264:1145-1148.

Lois C., Garcia-Verdugo J. M., Alvarez-Buylla A. (1996) Chain migration of neuronal precursors. *Science* 271:978-981.

Luskin M. B. (1993) Restricted proliferation and migration of postnatally generated neurons derived from the forebrain subventricular zone. *Neuron* 11:173-189.

Menn B., Garcia-Verdugo J M., Yaschine C., Gonzalez-Perez O., Rowitch D., Alvarez-Buylla A. (2006) Origin of oligodendrocytes in the subventricular zone of the adult brain. *J Neurosci* 26:7907-7918.

Mercier F., Kitasako J. T., Hatton G. I. (2002) Anatomy of the brain neurogenic zones revisited: fractones and the fibroblast/macrophage network. *J Comp Neurol* 451:170-188.

Merkle F. T., Mirzadeh Z., Alvarez-Buylla A. (2007) Mosaic organization of neural stem cells in the adult brain. *Science* 317:381-384.

Merkle F. T., Tramontin A. D., Garcia-Verdugo J. M., Alvarez-Buylla A. (2004) Radial glia give rise to adult neural stem cells in the subventricular zone. *Proc Natl Acad Sci USA* 101:17528-17532.

Mirzadeh Z., Merkle F. T., Soriano-Navarro M., Garcia-Verdugo J. M., Alvarez-Buylla A. (2008) Neural stem cells confer unique pinwheel architecture to the ventricular surface in neurogenic regions of the adult brain. *Cell Stem Cell* 3:265-278.

Morshead C. M., Garcia A. D., Sofroniew M. V., van Der Kooy D. (2003) The ablation of glial fibrillary acidic protein-positive cells from the adult central nervous system results in the loss of forebrain neural stem cells but not retinal stem cells. *Eur J Neurosci* 18:76-84.

Morshead C. M., Reynolds B. A., Craig C. G., McBurney M. W., Staines W. A., Morassutti D., Weiss S., Van der Kooy D. (1994) Neural stem cells in the adult mammalian forebrain: A relatively quiescent subpopulation of subependymal cells. *Neuron* 13:1071-1082.

Pérez-Cañellas M. R., García-Verdugo J. M. (1996) Adult neurogenesis in the telencephalon of a lizard: A [$^3$H]thymidine autoradiographic and bromodeoxyuridine immunocytochemical study. *DevBrain Res* 93:49-61.

Quinones-Hinojosa A., Sanai N., Soriano-Navarro M., Gonzalez-Perez O., Mirzadeh Z., Gil-Perotin S., Romero-Rodriguez R., Berger M. S., Garcia-Verdugo J. M., Alvarez-Buylla A. (2006) Cellular composition and cytoarchitecture of the adult human subventricular zone: a niche of neural stem cells. *J Comp Neurol* 494:415-434.

Reynolds B., Weiss S. (1992) Generation of neurons and astrocytes from isolated cells of the adult mammalian central nervous system. *Science* 255:1707-1710.

Reznikov K. Y. (1991) Cell proliferation and cytogenesis in the mouse hippocampus. *Adv Anat Embryol Cell Biol* 122:1-74.

Rietze R. L., Valcanis H., Brooker G. F., Thomas T., Voss A. K., Bartlett P. F. (2001) Purification of a pluripotent neural stem cell from the adult mouse brain. *Nature* 412:736-739.

Sanai N., Tramontin A. D., Quinones-Hinojosa A., Barbaro N. M., Gupta N., Kunwar S., Lawton M. T., McDermott M. W., Parsa A. T., Manuel-Garcia Verdugo J., Berger M. S., Alvarez-Buylla A. (2004) Unique astrocyte ribbon in adult human brain contains neural stem cells but lacks chain migration. *Nature* 427:740-744.

Seaberg R. M., van der Kooy D. (2002) Adult rodent neurogenic regions: the ventricular subependyma contains neural stem cells, but the dentate gyrus contains restricted progenitors. *J Neurosci* 22:1784-1793.

Seri B., Garcia-Verdugo J. M., McEwen B. S., Alvarez-Buylla A. (2001) Astrocytes give rise to new neurons in the adult mammalian hippocampus. *J Neurosci* 21:7153-7160.

Shen Q., Wang Y., Kokovay E., Lin G., Chuang S. M., Goderie S. K., Roysam B., Temple S. (2008) Adult SVZ stem cells lie in a vascular niche: a quantitative analysis of niche cell-cell interactions. *Cell Stem Cell* 3:289-300.

Song H. J., Stevens C. F., Gage F. H. (2002) Neural stem cells from adult hippocampus develop essential properties of functional CNS neurons. *Nat Neurosci* 5:438-445.

Spassky N., Merkle F. T., Flames N., Tramontin A. D., Garcia-Verdugo J. M., Alvarez-Buylla A. (2005) Adult ependymal cells are postmitotic and are derived from radial glial cells during embryogenesis. *J Neurosci* 25:10-18.

Tavazoie M., Van der Veken L., Silva-Vargas V., Louissaint M., Colonna L., Zaidi B., Garcia-Verdugo J. M., Doetsch F. (2008) A specialized vascular niche for adult neural stem cells. *Cell Stem Cell* 3:279-288.

Vescovi A. L., Reynolds B. A., Fraser D. D., Weiss S. (1993) bFGF regulates the proliferative fate of unipotent (neuronal) and bipotent (neuronal/astroglial) EGF-generated CNS progenitor cells. *Neuron* 11: 951-966.

Weiss S., Reynolds B. A., Vescovi A. L., Morshead C., Craig C. G., Van der Kooy D. (1996) Is there a neural stem cell in the mammalian forebrain? *Trends Neurosci* 19:387-393.

Wichterle H., Garcia-Verdugo J. M., Alvarez-Buylla A. (1997) Direct evidence for homotypic, glia-independent neuronal migration. *Neuron* 18:779-791.

In: Astrocytes
Editor: Oscar González-Pérez
ISBN: 978-1-62081-558-8
© 2012 Nova Science Publishers, Inc.

*Chapter V*

# Ultrastructural Characteristics of Astrocytic Neural Stem Cells in the Adult Brain

*Irene Sanchez-Vera[1,]\*, Arantxa Cebrian-Silla[2,]\*,
M. Salome Sirerol-Piquer,[1]
and Jose Manuel Garcia-Verdugo[1,2,#]*

[1]Laboratorio de Morfologia Celular, Centro de Investigacion Principe Felipe, CIBERNED, Avda, Valencia, Spain
[2]Laboratorio de Neurobiologia Comparada, Instituto Cavanilles de Biodiversidad y Biología Evolutiva, Universidad de Valencia, Valencia, Spain

## Abstract

During embryonic development neuroepithelial cells from the primordial ventricular system or ventricular zone (VZ) transform into radial glial cells. These cells give rise to neurons and glia during brain development. Radial glial cells are observed postnatally and during adulthood at least in two brain areas: the subventricular zone (SVZ) at lateral walls of the lateral ventricles, and the subgranular zone (SGZ) of the dentate gyrus of the hippocampus. These cells are astrocytes, type B cells or neural stem cells (NSCs) due to their capacity to divide and produce neurons, oligodendrocytes and astrocytes. The SVZ and the SGZ are conserved in mammals from rodents to humans, although the organization of NSCs and their progeny differs slightly among species. Moreover, in all species analyzed, NSCs present astrocytic nature. In the SVZ, astrocytes or type B cells are characterized by the presence of glial fibrillaryacidic protein (GFAP) intermediate filaments as well as their irregular nuclear contours. Some of these cells extend expansions and contact the blood vessels (astrocytic endfeet). Structurally, there are two subtypes of B cells: subtype B1 cells, contact the lumen of the ventricle exhibiting a short

---

\* Irene Sanchez-Vera and Arantxa Cebrian-Silla contributed equally to this work.
# Correspondenceto: Jose Manuel Garcia-Verdugo, Departamento de Neurobiologia Comparada, Instituto Cavanilles, Universidad de Valencia. C) Catedratico Jose Beltran N°2, CP: 46980, Paterna, Valencia, Spain. E-mail: j.manuel.garcia@uv.es.

single cilium (primary cilium) and subtype B2 cells, which do not contact the ventricle, are smaller and send the primary cilium to the underlying parenchyma. Evidence points type B1 cells as the NSCs. While in rodents the SVZ is a unique discontinuous region or layer containing the astrocytes, as well as their progeny. In primates, including human, astrocytes appear arranged in the ribbon astrocyte layer composed by their cell bodies, which is separated from the ependymal cell layer by the GAP layer, mainly composed ependymal and astrocytic expansions. In the rodent hippocampus, astrocytes or type B locate at the SGZ. Similarly to the SVZ, structurally there are two subtypes of astrocytes: radial astrocytes that present a GFAP-enriched radial process that cross the granular cell layer and horizontal astrocytes, which display horizontally along the SGZ and do not present the radial process. Type B cells divide and produce type D cells and neuroblasts. These structural units are known as hippocampal neurogenic niches. Although is widely accepted the existence of NSCs in SGZ of primates and humans the existence and characterization of neurogenic niches is poorly described. In this chapter we present a detailed ultrastructural description of the NSCs and the germinative areas, the SVZ and the SGZ, in rodents, primates and humans.

**Keywords**: Neural stem cells, subventricular zone, subgranular zone, astrocytes, ultrastructure, glial fibrillary acidic protein, proliferation, rodent, non-human primates and human

## Introduction

Since the early 100s, it has been generally believed that the adult central nervous system (CNS) of mammals has very limited regenerative capacity [1]. However, almost five decades ago, pioneering work by Altman & Das suggested continuing neurogenesis throughout adulthood in rodents [2], and since the early 1990, a large body of work has demonstrated that new neurons are indeed born in restricted regions of the adult mammalian CNS, the subventricular zone (SVZ) of the lateral ventricles and the subgranular zone (SGZ) of the dentate gyrus (DG) in the hippocampus [3-5] (Figure 1). Both areas contain neural stem cells (NSCs), which have the ability to self-renew and to give rise to the three major cell types in the CNS: neurons, astrocytes and oligodendrocytes [4]. Moreover, other regions with proliferative capacity have been identified, such as the third and fourth ventricle, the spinal cord and the hypothalamus. However, there is no evidence that this proliferation give rise to new neurons under normal conditions. The identity of neural stem cells that give rise to new neurons in the adult CNS has been a subject of hot debate for the past few years. Several cell types have been proposed as the resident adult NSCs, including astrocytes [6] and multiciliated ependymal cells [7] although the astrocyte hypothesis is currently the most accepted. The addition of new neurons throughout life raises the exciting possibility that stimulation of this process can be applied as a new strategy for therapy for CNS diseases that had hitherto been thought intractable [8, 9]. In this chapter we review the current knowledge of NSCs. We first summarize their origin and then we focus our attention on the histological and ultrastructural characterization of NSCs in the SVZ and DG of different species including rodent, non-human primates and human.

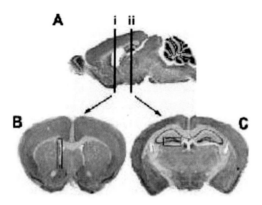

Figure 1. Illustrative images of the proliferative areas in the rodent brain. (A) Nissl-stained mouse sagital section with two different levels indicating the SVZ (i) and the dentate gyrus of hippocampus (ii). (B) Coronal section at level i showing the SVZ in squared areas. (C) Coronal section at level ii showing the dentate gyrus of the hippocampus. Images taken from brainmaps.org website.

## Origin of Neural Stem Cells (NSCs)

Central nervous system (CNS) development is an intricate process relying on a series of mechanisms precisely regulated in time and space. The CNS begins as a sheet made up of primary progenitors known as neuroepithelial cells (NE). The edges of this epithelial sheet fold together to form the neural tube. The core of primitive brain, which is filled with fluid, will become later the ventricular system and the spinal canal. In mice, at embryonic day (E) eight, NE are radially elongated and contact both the apical (ventricular) and basal (pial) surfaces, forming the ventricular zone (VZ). Although the VZ is composed of a single layer of NE, the neuroephitelium looks pseudostratified, because of the characteristic alternate movement of the nucleus between the basal and the apical surface (interkinetic nuclear migration) [10]. This migration is synchronized with the cell cycle: at mitosis, the nucleus stands at the apical surface, near the ventricle, moving towards the basalsurface during phase G1, reaching the most basal location in S phase, and then migrating back apically during the G2 phase.

Initially, NE divide symmetrically to increase the pool of stem cells [11, 12]. After expansion, NE start to divide asymmetrically, giving rise to another NE and either to a neuron or, alternatively, to an intermediate progenitor cell (IPC) or basal progenitor, which migrates basally and divide symmetrically to produce neurons and glia [13-15]. IPC or basal progenitors form a layer at the border between the VZ and the pre-plate, known as the subventricular zone (SVZ). With the switch to neurogenesis (around E9-10 in mice), NE down-regulate certain epithelial features and begin to transform into radial glial cells (RG). RG remain in contact with both pial and ventricular surfaces, their cell bodies are retained within the VZ [16]. RG are characterized by their soma orthogonally elongated to the VZ contacting the ventricle lumen, where they extend a single primary cilium. By one hand, their cytoplasm contains abundant organelle, mainly the smooth endoplasmic reticulum and intermediate filaments arrange aligned along the long axis of the cell. By other hand, the nuclei appear elongated and profusely invaginated. It contains lax chromatin and one or two nucleoli [17]. As the thickness of the nervous tissue increases with the generation of large numbers of neurons, the basal process (pial-directed radial processes) of the RG elongates in order to retain attachment to the pial surface [18]. These morphological changes are accompanied by the acquisition of 25-nm microtubules and 9-nm intermediate filaments within the radial fiber, [19-21]. The RG cells also begin to express astroglial markers such as the astrocyte-specific glutamate transporter (GLAST), brain lipid-binding protein (BLBP), and Tenascin C (TN-C) (for review, see Campbell and Gotz 2002 [22]). They also express a variety of intermediate filament proteins including Nestin, Vimentin, the RC1 and RC2 epitopes [23], and in some species the astroglial intermediate filament, glial fibrillary acidic protein (GFAP) [20, 24, 25]. At about the same time, the tight junctional complexes that couple neuroepithelial cells convert to adherens junctions [26, 27], and the cells begin to make astrocyte-like specialized contact with endothelial cells of the developing cerebral vasculature [28-30].

Radial glia cell bodies reside in the VZ throughout the period of cortical development, participating in neurogenesis and guiding neuronal migration. At the end of this developmental period, most RG cells lose their ventricular attachment and migrate toward the cortical plate by a process of somal translocation. In mammals, most RG cells transform into astrocytes [20, 28, 31]. The morphology of RG changes from bipolar spanning the cortex to unipolar that no longer contacts the ventricle to multipolar with a regressing radial process, thus progressively taking on astrocytic morphology. Moreover, the disappearance of RG is coincident with the appearance of increasing numbers of astrocytes [28, 32]. However, a subset of RG known as type B cells, astrocytes or NSCs persist postnatally mainly in two regions the subventricular zone (SVZ) of the lateral wall of the lateral ventricle and the subgranular zone of the dentate gyrus (DG) of the hippocampus, and are able also to give rise neurons, astrocytes and oligodendrocytes. These two brain regions persist among mammalian species from rodent to human [30].

## Subventricular Zone Cellular Organization

Early in the last century, Allen identified mitotic cells in the SVZ of the lateral wall of the lateral ventricle in adult rats [33]. Proliferating cells persist in the SVZ of many adult vertebrates, including dogs [34], rabbits [35], rodents [36, 37], primates [38, 39] and human [40-43]. In this chapter we will review the ultrastructural features of adult NSCs in rodents, non-human primates and humans.

### Neural Stem Cells in Rodent Lateral Ventricles

The SVZ has been widely described in rodents, especially in mouse. In the mouse brain, the SVZ is located close to the striatum and the lateral wall of the lateral ventricles (Figure 1A, B). The SVZ is a source of neural stem cells (NSCs) for brain areas such as the corpus callosum and the olfactory bulb [44, 45]. The SVZ is a thin discontinuous layer, formed from one to four cell layers [42]. It is physically limited by the ependymal layer in contact to the lateral ventricles although some data show SVZ astrocytes (type B cells) beside the ependymal cells [46] (Figure 2A, B and F).

Four cell types, with several subtypes, have been described in the SVZ: migrating neuroblasts (type A), immature precursors (type C), astrocytes (type B) subdivided in B1 and B2 subtypes and ependymal cells (type E) with E1 and E2 subtypes. The migrating neuroblasts (type A cells) advance as chains through tubes defined by the processes of slowly proliferating SVZ astrocytes (type B). These clusters of rapidly dividing immature precursors (type C cells) are scattered along the network of migrating chains [47] (Figure 2A, B and F). Numerous experiments concluded that type B cells are the NSCs in the adult SVZ. Type B cells divide to give rise to type C cells, which in turn divide repeatedly, forming tight clusters that then generate type A cells [48].

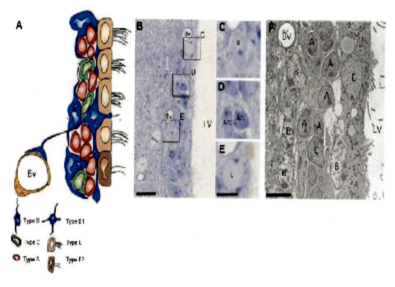

Figure 2. Cell composition and organization in the mouse SVZ. (A) Illustrative representation of different cell types, their relation with blood vessels and the cytoarchitecture in the SVZ. (B-E) Toluidine-blue stained SVZ semithin section (1.5µm). B) Panoramic view of SVZ, where squared areas show different cell types. C) High magnification of type B cell. D) Cell type with shared features between type C and A cells. E) Ependymal cell (type E cell). (F) SVZ ultrathin section (60-70nm) indicating the different cells types and their organization. Scale-bar: B=10µm; C, D and E=5µm and F=5µm. Bv=blood vessel, LV=lateral ventricle, B=type B cell, E=ependymal cell, A=type A cell and C=type C cell.

At light microscope (LM), SVZ cells show different features, which allow us to distinguish them. Type B cells (neural stem cell) are larger and irregular with light and invaginated nuclei. Depending on the amount of intermediate filaments, the cytosol can be light or dark although always less dark than type A cells (Figure 2A-C). They can appear scattered but also form small clusters in the boundaries of type A cells. At LM we cannot distinguish between the subtypes B1 and B2 cells although we know that B1 cells are located between the ependymal cells and the ventricular lumen, and B2 cells are in the parenchyma. The morphology of type B cells depends on the surrounding environment hence the study of neighboring cells is also relevant to understand the NSCs and the SVZ function. Type A cells (migratory neuroblasts) are smaller and darker forming clusters close to the ventricle (Figure 2A, B and D). Type C cells (transient amplifying cells) are the most complex to identify in the LM due to their shared features with A and B cells. Type C cells are found in the close vicinity of type Acells (Figure 2A, B and E). Type E cells (ependymal cells) are cubical or columnar shaped lining the cavity of the lateral ventricle. They possess cilia in their apical pole and lipid drops within their cytosol. The nuclei are round or oval (Figure 2A-B). Subtype E1 and E2 cells cannot be distinguished at LM.

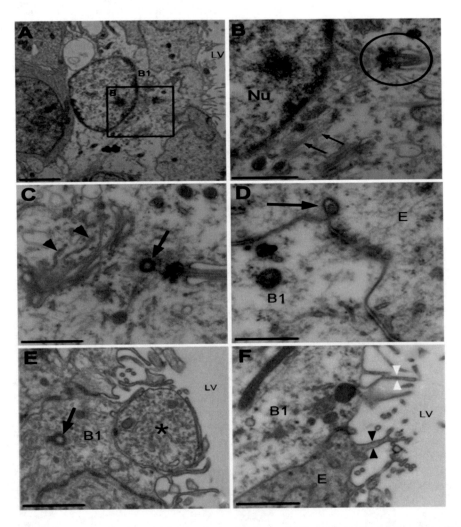

Figure 3. Ultrastructural features of type B1 cells in the mouse SVZ. (A)Type B1 cell present a light cytoplasm and a single primary cilium in contact with the ventricle. (B) Higher magnification detail of squared area in A image, with basal body of the cilium (circle), intermediated filaments in the cytoplasm (arrows), and clumps of chromatin in the nucleus. (C) Detail of the RER (black arrowheads) and the centriole perpendicular to the basal body (arrow). (D) Endocytic phenomena (arrow) between a type B1 and an ependymal cell. (E) Type B1 cell, (containing the centriole; arrow), in contact with a ventricular axon (asterisk). The axon presents vesicles. Microvilli of type B1 and ependymal cells sheath the axon (asterisk). (F) Detail of ependymal (black arrowheads) and type B1 (white arrowheads) microvilli. Microvilli of type B1 cells appear thinner and longer than ependymal microvilli. Scale-bar: A=2µm; B and C=1µm; D=500nm and E and F=1µm. LV=lateral ventricle, B1=type B1 cell, E=ependymal cell, * =axon and Nu=Nucleus.

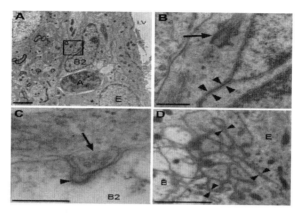

Figure 4. Ultrastructural features of type B2 cells in the mouse SVZ. (A) Panoramic view of a type B2 cell that presents a primary cilium directed to the underlying parenchyma and the inner nuclear membrane fusion. (B) Higher magnification detail of the primary cilium (arrow) and the inner nuclear membrane fusion (black arrowheads). (C) Detail of an endocytic vesicle coated by clathrin (arrowhead) with its own primary cilium (arrow) in a type B2 cell. (D) Branched fractones (arrowheads) contacting type B and ependymal cells to increase the contact cell surface. Scale-bar: A=2µm; B=500nm; C=200nm and D=2µm. B2=type B2 cell, LV=lateral ventricle, B=type B cell and E=ependymal cell.

At electron microscopy (EM) the different cell types are more easily recognizable (Figure 2F) albeit sometimes their identification is especially complex in the transitional stages between different cell types. Ultrastructurally type B cells have irregular contours that profusely fill the spaces between neighboring cells. Cytoplasm is lighter with few ribosomes and enriched in intermediate filaments (Figure 3A, B). Golgi apparatus and rough endoplasmic reticulum (RER) do not form Nissl bodies. However, we can find two-three parallel cisternae of RER. The dictiosomes are often associated to basal bodies of cilia (Figure 3C). Frequently these cells have a deeply invaginated nucleus with clumps of dense chromatin (Figure 3A, B). Type B cell-astrocytes establish cell-to-cell contact with other astrocytes and ependymal cells through gap junctions and adherent junctions. Astrocytes also establish adherent junctions but no gap junctions with type C cells or migratory neuroblasts. These cells constitute a dense network underlying the ependymal layer and surround the chains of type A cells. Type B cells, in contact with other cell types (type B, C, A and E cells), can show endocytic phenomena of the cell membrane (Figure 3D and 4C). These 'bites' of membrane can be filled of extracellular matrix or the cytoplasm of the neighboring cell. In aged rodents, electrodense bodies and lipofucsine granules are accumulated within the cytoplasm of type B cells.

The above-described features are frequent characteristics of type B cells albeit depending on metabolic changes or cell differentiation stages we can observe some heterogeneity. In adult mice two types of B cells were described, type B1 and B2. Type B1 sends a short primary cilium (Figure 3A-B) that contacts the lumen of the ventricle, and has less organelles in their cytoplasm than type B2 cells. Type B1 cells have also microvilli contacting with the ventricle lumen but longer and thinner than those in ependymal cells (Figure 3F). Type B1 cells contact with ependymal cells through long junctional complexes without altering their cell morphology, other astrocytes, type C and A cells. They also establish contact with blood vessels through long and thin expansions (endfeet) [49] and with axons in the ventricle lumen.

Three-dimensional reconstructions in B1 cells show a perpendicular orientated centriole to basal bodies (Figure 3C). Unlike ependymal cells, the basal bodies of B1 cells are at a minimum distance of 1 µm from the cell surface. However, if the contact of B1 cell surface with the ventricle lumen is lower, the distance from the basal bodies to the cell membrane will be shorter. We can find axons, whose origin is currently unknown, in the ventricular lumen. The axons contain abundant microtubules and vesicles. The vesicles can be light or dark with round-to-pleomorphic morphology (Figure 3E). The types of neurotransmitters filling the vesicles are unknown. The axons occasionally show bulbous processes contacting with type B1 and ependymal cells. Microvilli of both cell types surround the axons as a sheath, which could be anchoring the axons to the ventricular surface at certain locations (Figure 3E). Unlike B1 cells, B2 astrocytes do not contact with the lumen of the ventricle and their short primary cilium directs to the underlying parenchyma. Type B2 astrocytes are smaller and have clumped chromatin, a scarce cytosol with more organelles and tend to localize at the interface with the striatal parenchyma (Figure 4A, B). Type B2 cells have also more outstanding intermediate filaments than type B1 cells. Intermediate filaments are found in the expansions, far from the cell body. Type B2 cells have one-two nucleoli. Around 40% of type B cells (mostly type B2 cells) show one-two fusions of their inner nuclear membrane with a rod-like appearance (Figure 4A, B). This phenomenon is frequent in type B cells albeit rarely can also be observed in ependymal, migratory cells and in cells sharing some features of C cells which could correspond to a transitional stage between B and C cell. Occasionally we can observe clathrin-coated vesicles at the cell membrane that sheathes its own cilium (Figure 4C). The biological sense of this phenomenon is unknown. In the septum, there are only type B2 astrocytes constituting a thin monolayer that separates ependymal cells from the underlying neuropile [50]. Unlike type B1 cells, type B2 cells do not establish junctional complexes with the ependymal cells albeit occasionally we can observe small adherent junctions. Astrocyte cells surround neuroblasts and can isolate the ependyma from neuropile forming a thin bound between both. Astrocytes, mainly type B2 cells, directly contact to a novel type of extracellular matrix called as fractones. Fractones have a branched morphology allows each fracton to directly contact numerous type B cells and other cells of the ventricle wall. By their electrodensity, fractones resemble basement membranes (basal laminae) [51, 52] (Figure 4D). Fractones contain proteoglycans that collect, concentrate and activate growth factors as FGF2 being essential for activating FGF2 at the neural stem cell surface [53].

In the embryonic VZ, the primary neural progenitors are radial glia [15]. After birth, from P0 to P7, radial glia transform into parenchymal astrocytes [54] and ependymal cells [55] contacting both cell types with the ventricular lumen. Astrocytes possess a single, short cilium with a perpendicular orientated centriole. Ependymal cells are multiciliated and, at this stage, the basal bodies of cilia are being assembled. Monociliated cells have an electrodense cytoplasm with large Golgi apparatus, abundant organelles, mitochondria and ribosomes. These cells show inner nuclear membrane fusions as in the adult stage.

Ependymal cells progressively, from P15 to P30, populate the walls of the lateral ventricle [56]. Monociliated cells (astrocytes) have a lighter cytoplasm with scarce organelles. Progressively the number or ventricle-contacting astrocytes decreases with age. In the adult, primary progenitors have been identified as a subpopulation of B1 astrocytes [6], which are derived from radial glia. Radial glia cells send a long expansion that interacts with blood vessels [57]. Ventricle-contacting B1 cells undergo mitosis [58] as at embryonic stages although this phenomenon has not been observed at EM. Type B2 cells are also radial glia-derived [56] albeit there are no enough evidences establishing the cellular events during the development.

Unlike B cells, type A cells have an electrodense cytoplasm in the EM and characteristic intercellular spaces (Figure 2E). Type A cells are fusiform with one or two processes. The cytosol is scarce with a large number of free ribosomes, a few short cisternae of RER, small Golgi apparatus and many microtubules oriented along the axis of the cells while type B cells are devoid of microtubules within their cytoplasm. The plasma membrane displays characteristic junctional complexes with neighbor cells. The nucleus is dark, occasionally invaginated without inner nuclear membrane fusions. Chromatin is mainly euchromatin with two-to-four small nucleoli.

Type C cells (transit amplifying precursors) share some features with the type A cells but they are more electrolucent, have fewer ribosomes, and they are not found in the RMS. Their cytoplasm contains a large Golgi apparatus and no bundles of intermediate filaments or microtubules. Their nuclei are larger, spherical and frequently invaginated with rare inner nuclear fusions and several nucleoli [50]. Both type A and C cells have proliferative activity albeit they have not been identified as neural stem cells.

Finally, type E cells (ependymal cells) are large and cubical and they physically form a monolayer that separates the lateral ventricle from the surrounding parenchyma (Figure 2F). A main feature of these cells is the presence of multiple cilia and numerous microvilli in the apical pole of the cell. Ependymal cells do not have centriole. The lateral processes are interspersed between contiguous cells and remain in close contact through many junctional complexes such as tight junctions and desmosomes. The cytosol of type E cells is electrolucent with few organelles and, unlike type B cells, contains abundant mitochondria. The nucleus is round-to-oval shaped, composed of sparse chromatin with clusters of heterochromatin associated with the nuclear membrane. In the basal pole, some cells send an expansion that interacts with the basal lamina of blood vessels. Within the cytoplasm of ependymal cells smaller amount of intermediate filaments can be observed in rodents than in higher mammals (human or non-human primate).

In mice two subtypes of ependymal cells has been described: subtype E1 cells, with multiple basal bodies and multiple long cilia, and subtype E2 cells with two long cilia and complex, pinwheel-shaped basal bodies. In E1 cells mitochondria are bound to the base of the cilia through filamentous structures while in E2 cells mitochondria are concentrated around the nucleus.

Other cell types can be sporadically found in the SVZ such as neurons, pyknotic cells, oligodendrocytes, and microglia mixed up with the described populations [50].

We can also observe some mitosis in cells with dark and light cytoplasm corresponding to type A and C cells, and type B cells respectively.

## Neural Stem Cells in Non-human Primate Lateral Ventricles

Multipotential progenitors have been identified in the postnatal SVZ of the primate forebrain [59]. In non-human primates, the SVZ is composed of three layers: ependymal, hypocellular, and astrocytic cell layer (Figure 5A). The ependymal cells (Vimentin-positive) forms a monolayer of cubical cells and in some portions of the SVZ can be flat (ventral wall of the temporal region). The ependymal cells send expansions to the neuropile while in mice we can find thin expansions parallel and perpendicular orientated to the ependymal surface.

The hypocellular layer, absent in rodents, is devoid of cell bodies and is composed almost exclusively of astrocytic and ependymal expansions (Vimentin and GFAP +) with variable thicknesses. This layer is located between the ependyma and the astrocytic cell layer.

The bodies of the astrocytes form a ribbon of astrocytic cell bodies that runs along the SVZ in parallel with the ependymal layer [60]. Several types of astrocyte-like cells have been observed in the SVZ.

All of them share as features intermediate filaments distributed in both, the soma and the cell expansions and an irregularly shaped, invaginated nucleus but to a lesser extent than those in mice. Occasionally we can observe inner nuclear membrane fusions similar to those previously described in mice (Figure 5C, D).

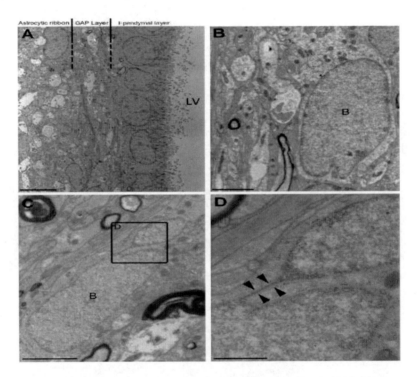

Figure 5. Ultrastructural details and organization of the non-human primates SVZ. (A) Panoramic view of the SVZ showing the ependymal, GAP and astrocytic ribbon layer. (B) Detail of type B cells with light cytoplasm. (C) Detail of type B cells with dark cytoplasm. (D) Higher magnification detail of squared area in C image. The nucleus presents an inner nuclear membrane fusion (arrowheads). Scale-bar: A=5μm; B=2.5μm; C=2μm and D=500nm. LV=lateral ventricle.

The most abundant astrocyte is mainly found in the ribbon layer. These astrocytes have electrodense cytoplasm with abundant organelles and intermediate filaments. These astrocytes are called as DB (dark type B cells) in *Macaca fascicularis* and B2 cells in *Callithrix jacchus* (marmoset). Both DB and B2 cells are essential elements of the astrocyte ribbon layer. Occasionally their cytoplasm contains lysosomal bodies. Their nuclei morphology can vary depending on the cytoplasm processes. The nuclei contain one or two reticulated, oval nucleoli and lax chromatin with some clumps at the inner nuclear membrane. These astrocytes have cytoplasmatic extensions that project into the GAP layer. In *M. fascicularis* we can also distinguish, in the ribbon layer, type LB astrocytes (light type B cells) with fewer intermediate filaments and more organelles within their cytosol. LB and DB astrocytes are in direct contact with the basal lamina of the blood vessels. Only in marmoset have been described type B1 astrocytes in contact with the ventricle displaying a single, short cilium with a perpendicularly orientated centriole [61]. Both LB and B1 cells are close to the cavity of lateral ventricle although not always contacting to the ventricular lumen [60, 61]. The astrocytes at the ribbon layer occasionally divide. New neurons tend to organize in chain-like structures, which are surrounded by astrocytes. These chain-like structures are immersed in the GAP layer of the SVZ and in the RMS. This pattern is highly reminiscent of that observed in rodent RMS, but not in adult humans [60]. Migratory neuroblasts (type A cells) are fusiform and often bipolar. In the SVZ, type A cells form clusters of cells with intercellular spaces surrounded by cytoplasmatic expansions of the ependymal cells and astrocytes. The neuroblasts are elongated and show a sparse dark cytoplasm and microtubule-rich processes. Nuclei are oval, rarely invaginated, and are composed of clusters of heterochromatin and large nucleoli [60, 61].

Type C cells are not described in non-human primates although in marmoset, a cell type with mixed morphological features of astrocytes and neuroblast has been identified. We hypothesize that this cell type is equivalent to rodent type C or precursor cells. These cells are large and display long cytoplasm extensions. Their cytoplasm is dark, rich in microtubules, and contains mostly mitochondria, RER, and free ribosomes. The nucleus is large, with deep invaginations, and lax chromatin [61].

Ependymal cells (type E cells) are cubical-cylindrical epithelial cells that layer the ventricles. These cells are multiciliated (9+2) and have abundant microvilli in their apical side. Mitochondria are abundant and especially related to the basal body of the cilia. The nucleus is oval and mainly composed of euchromatin with clusters of heterochromatin at the inner nuclear membrane. Ependymal cells send long radial expansions towards the neuropile. We can find some ependymal-like cells within the GAP layer displaying the above-described features. The function of this displaced ependyma is currently unknown albeit it has been suggested that it could have a relevant role during the development by increasing the contact surface of type B cells with cerebrospinal fluid. Unlike rodents, in non-human primates, ependymal E2 type has not been described [60, 61].

## Neural Stem Cells in Human Lateral Ventricles

In the mid-1990s human SVZ explants derived from temporal lobectomies in patients with refractory epilepsy were utilized to demonstrate that the adult human forebrain was capable of *in vitro* neuronal production [41, 62]. Few years later, adult cancer patients were infused with BrdU to label mitotically active cells. BrdU-positive cells were found within the SVZ demonstrating that cells with proliferative capacity are present throughout life [40].

In humans, the SVZ is located in the lateral wall of the lateral ventricles and host cells with astrocytic features that proliferate. Isolation and *in vitro* culture of SVZ-derived astrocytes demonstrated their self-renewing and multipotency abilities giving rise to neurons, astrocytes, and oligodendrocytes. These studies concluded that astrocytes are the adult neural stem cells in human [43]. The cytoarchitecture of the SVZ in humans is similar to that previously described in non-human primates. It can be divided in three distinct layers varying in thickness and cell density: [1] a unique layer composed of cubical ependymal cells in touch with the ventricular lumen. These cells send radial expansions into the glial network (neuropile) and the second layer, [2] a hypocellular layer or GAP layer with fewer cells, basically formed by a large number of ependymal and astrocytic expansions. GAP layer is thicker in humans than in non-human primates. Finally, [3] astrocyte ribbon layer is mainly composed of astrocytes bodies that send expansions to the GAP layer. This layer is constituted by large astrocytes, myelinic axons, and infrequent oligodendrocytes and displaced ependymal cells. These ependymal cells do not face the ventricles but form small clusters [43, 63]. The astrocytes express GFAP and Vimentin molecular markers [50]. At LM ependymal cells and astrocytes cannot be distinguished hence EM analysis is needed. Unfortunately, to collect well-preserved human SVZ samples are rare which makes difficult to analyze their ultrastructural features at EM. Ultrastructurally, three astrocytic types are distinguished at the EM called as type B1, B2 and B3 cells. We want to note that the terminology used to classify type B cells does not correspond to the criteria applied in mice.

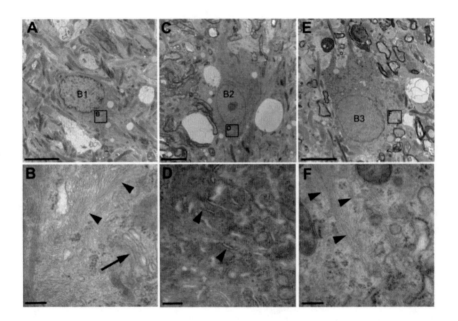

Figure 6. Ultrastructural features of astrocytes in the human SVZ. (A) Panoramic view of a type B1 cell. (B) Higher magnification detail of squared area in A image. Cytoplasm containing dense bundles of long intermediate filaments (arrowheads) and large Golgi apparatus (arrow). (C) Panoramic view of a type B2 cell with a large cell body. (D) Higher magnification detail of squared area in C image. Cytoplasm containing abundant RER cisternae (arrowheads). (E) Panoramic view of a type B3 cell presenting a large cell body. Higher magnification detail of squared area in E image. Cytoplasm presents organelles and intermediate filaments (arrowheads). Scale-bar: A, C and E=5μm; Band I=200nm; D=500nm and G=2μm. B1= type B1 astrocytes, B2=type B2 astrocytes and B3=type B3 astrocytes.

The first type is a small astrocyte (B1) with long, tangentially oriented horizontal projections. This is the predominant type of astrocyte in GAP layer. In comparison to mice and non-human primates, type B1 cells do not share as feature a primary cilium contacting to the ventricular lumen. Unlike type B2 and B3 cells, B1 cells have scarce cytoplasm with large Golgi apparatus and polyribosomes, dense bundles of long intermediate filaments and occasional lipid drops (Figure 6A-B). The second type of astrocyte (B2) is large and mainly found at the interface of the hypocellular layer and the ribbon of cells and within astrocyte ribbon layer. These astrocytes have large expansions, large cell bodies, and abundant organelles (mitochondria, intermediate filament, RER cisternae and endoplasmic reticulum vesicles) (Figure 6C-D) [63]. The third and last type of astrocyte (B3) is also large, but has few cytoplasmatic organelles and a much lighter cytoplasm [63]. B3 cells are mainly observed in the interface between the astrocyte ribbon layer and the surrounding neuropile (Figure 6E-F). Occasionally we can observe differences in the intensity of intermediate filaments because of the fixation or preservation of tissues (Figure 6G-I).

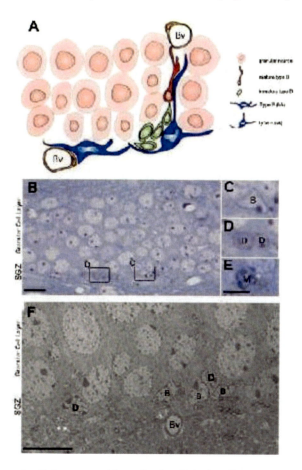

Figure 7. Organization and cellular composition of rodent DG. (A) Illustrative diagram of the cell composition and organization in the DG. (B-E) Coronal toluidine-blue stained semithin section (1.5μm) of rodent SGZ. B) Panoramic view of the DG, where squared areas show the different cell types. C) High magnification of a type B cell. D) Type D cells. E) Microglial cell. (F) Electron microscopy panoramic view, indicating the different cell types in the SGZ. Scale-bar: B=10μm; C, D and E=5μm and F=20μm. Bv=Blood vessels, B=type B cell, D=type D cell and M=microglial cell.

The cellular events of astrocytes during the postnatal development are unknown due to the lack of well-preserved human SVZ samples. However, it is reported that astrocytes of the ribbon cell layer increase their proliferative activity in patients with amyotrophic lateral sclerosis or after ischemic stroke [64, 65]. Processes from astrocytes, in the GAP layer, contain dense bundles of GFAP+ intermediate filaments, few organelles and some mitochondria, as well as small vesicles distributed along each expansion. Astrocytic processes form a remarkable network of interconnected processes joined to each other by gap junctions and large desmosomes. Gap junctions and desmosomes are also present along the soma of the few displaced astrocytes occasionally present in the hypocellular GAP [63]. Unlike rodents, the neuroblasts in the anterior SVZ and RMS, appear migrating isolated or in pairs [66], but never in chains [43]. These cells have only been identified using molecular markers but they have not been ultrastructurally characterized yet.

In the ependymal layer, ependymal cells are found to be cuboidal with round-to-oval nuclei, sparse chromatin, and 1–2 nucleoli. Their cytoplasm contains numerous organelles, unlike rodent ependymal cells, which possess far fewer. In the apical portion these cells have abundant microvilli and cilia that display a 9+2 microtubule organization. Laterally, the cells present numerous, deep interdigitations with other ependymal cells with desmosomes and tight junctions. Many of the ependymal cells have basal expansions oriented perpendicularly, away from the ventricle. Other expansions turn in the hypocellular GAP and run parallel to the ventricle wall. In comparison to astrocytes expansions, ependymal cell processes in the hypocellular GAP region have fewer intermediate filaments, abundant mitochondria and vesicles (endoplasmic reticulum), and occasional lipofucsine granules [63].

Interestingly, cell bodies of ependymal cells can be found within GAP layer. They have been observed in young and old humans. Displaced ependymal cells form small round-oval rosettes containing 4–14 cells surrounding a central complex containing abundant microvilli, cilia, and junctional complexes. Their cilia contain a 9+2 microtubule organization. Furthermore, some displaced ependymal cells have short processes [63].

### *Hippocampal Neurogenesis*

The other region considered to be neurogenic in adult mammals is the dentate gyrus (DG) of the hippocampus. Although we talk about neurogenesis in the hippocampus, it should be noted that neurogenesis occurs only in the dentate gyrus (DG).

In the adult mammalian DG, NSCs reside in the so-called subgranular zone (SGZ), a rim band of tissue between the GCL and the hilus (Figure 7A). NSCs proliferate and newborn neurons in the SGZ migrate only a short distance to the granular cell layer (GCL), where they extend dendrites to the molecular layer and an axon along the mossy fiber pathway and integrate functionally into the circuitry of the dentate gyrus, becoming mature functional granule neurons [67-70].

Some authors point out the importance of these newborn neurons in cognitive processes like learning and memory [71, 72].

### *Neural Stem Cells In Rodent Hippocampus*

Using the same approach with the GFAP-Gtva transgenic mice and Ara-C as in the identification of SVZ´s NSCs, Alvarez-Buylla´s group provided evidence that astrocytes or type B cells are the NSCs in the SGZ of the hippocampus [5]. Two types of NSCs or astrocytes can be identified in the SGZ according to their specific morphologies and expression of unique sets of molecular markers. Radial astrocytes (rA or type 1 cells) have a radial process spanning the entire GCL. These processes are oriented tangentially along the

SGZ, and send thin lateral processes intercalated extensively between granule neurons that isolate them from neuropile. Radial astrocytes are characterized by the expression of GFAP, the glutamate receptor GLAST, Nestin and the SRY-related HMG (high mobility group) box transcription factor SOX2, and rarely enter into cell cycle. Non-radial or horizontal astrocytes (hA or type 2 cells) have only short processes and can be divide in two subtypes; the type 2a cells, express Nestin and SOX2 but do not have the radial GFAP process, and enter into cell cycle more often [73-75] and type 2b that are SOX2+ quiescent stem cells [76]. It has been suggested that hA may arise from rA, but direct evidence delineating this lineage relationship is still lacking.

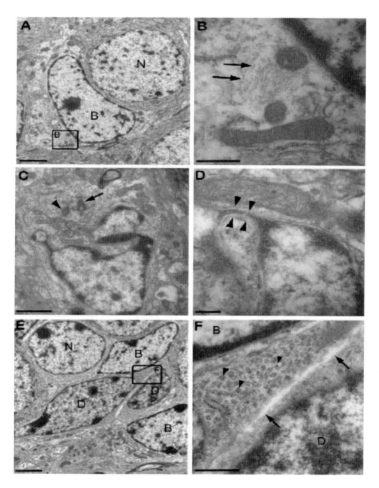

Figure 8. SGZ ultrastructural features. (A) Type B cell with light cytoplasm and characteristic irregular contours close to a granular neuron. (B) High magnification of squared area in A image, showing a dense network of intermediate filaments (arrows). (C) Type B cell with dark cytoplasm, elevated number of organelles, inner nuclear membrane fusions, and a primary cilium (arrow) with its centriole (arrow head). These morphological features have not been specifically associated to rA or hA. (D) Detail of a type B inner nuclear membrane fusion (arrowheads). (E) Panoramic view of a SGZ neurogenic niche composed of a couple of type B and D cells. (F) High magnification of squared area in E image. Cytoplasm of type D cell is dark, containing more polyribosomes than astrocytes (arrow heads) and the plasma membrane is smooth. Characteristic extracellular spaces are present between migrating cells and astrocytes (arrows). Scale-bar: A=2μm; B=500nm; C=1μm; D=200nm; E=2 μm and F=500nm. B=type B cell and D=type D cell.

Like in the SVZ, the SGZ NSC's function depends on the cell types that form this region. These cell types are type D cells, the intermediate precursors in the generation of new granular neurons in the dentate gyrus, microglia and endothelial cells that form the neurogenic niches and show different morphological and ultrastructural features, which allow us to distinguish them. Large gabaergic neurons can be also observed within the SGZ. At LM type B cells are characterized by an irregular and elongated nucleus with clumps of heterochromatin, and lighter cytoplasm than the other cell types in the SGZ. This cell type appears isolated or forming clusters of even tree cells and shows homogeneous distribution throughout the SGZ (Figure 7B-C). Analysis on semithin section (1.5µm) only allows a general description of type B cells in the SGZ, the reduced thickness makes very difficult, if not impossible, the differentiation between rA and hA. In the other hand, type D cells (migratory neuroblasts) have and spherical nucleus with dense chromatin, dark cytoplasmatic and nuclear matrix and do not present heterochromatin clumps, that contrast with type B cells (Figure 7B and D).

Microglial cells present dense euchromatin, big perinuclear clumps of heterochromatin and dark bodies in the cytoplasm, which differentiate them from the above cells types (type B and D cells). Microglial cells are located in the GL and in the SGZ, quite frequently associated to neurogenic niches (Figure 7B and E). At transmission electron microscopy these cell types are more easily recognized (Figure 7F), but like in the SVZ, sometimes the transitional stage between different cell types makes difficult its classification. Both types of astrocytes, rA and hA, can be distinguished, although occasionally tridimensional reconstructions are necessary. Radial astrocytes have a large cell body with a major radial process that penetrated the GCL. Tangentially oriented expansions along the SGZ and thin lateral processes from these astrocytes intercalated extensively between granule neurons are characterized by their pale cytoplasm containing mainly intermediate filaments and few organelles. The radial process branched profusely in the molecular layer (ML) and is enriched in GFAP intermediate filaments. In contrast, hAs had no radial projection, but instead extended branched processes parallel to the SGZ and thin short secondary branches into the hilus and the GCL. Horizontal astrocytes were generally elongated, whereas radial astrocytes had a round, polygonal, or triangular cell body. Both hAs and rAs had a light cytoplasm, a dense network of intermediate filaments (Figure 8A-B), irregularly shaped cell contours that intercalated between neighbouring cells, chromatin in granules, small Golgi apparatus and endoplasmic reticulum, darker mitochondria than neurons, were in contact with other astrocytes through gap junctions [74] and present a primary cilium, required to mediate stem/progenitors cell maintenance probably oriented towards the blood vessels (unpublished data) [77, 78]. Radial astrocytes had more organelles, polyribosomes, and lighter mitochondria compared with horizontal astrocytes. In addition, large bundles of intermediate filaments present in the main process of radial astrocytes were less prominent in hAs.

However, this radial and horizontal classification not always includes all SGZ astrocytes. This fact may be due to the morphological and molecular changes that astrocytes undergo at the process of generation new neurons or even astrocytes (8A, C). Some of these morphological aspects, that have not been associated to rA or hA, are the presence of inner nuclear membrane fusions, identical to those observed in the SVZ, as well as junction complexes (Figure 8C-D). Type D cells are ultrastructurally very different to astrocytes. Type D cells have a smooth plasma membrane, dark scant cytoplasm containing lighter mitochondria to that observed in astrocytes, many more polyribosomes than astrocytes but less than granule neurons and present the characteristic extracellular spaces of brain migrating cells with astrocytes and neurons (Figure E-F) [74]. Interestingly astrocytes emit thin expansions that tend to isolate the SGZ of the hilus and to ensheath type D cells, probably until they have some degree of maturity and begin to establish stable circuits.

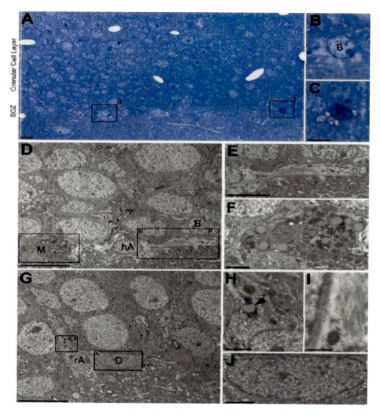

Figure 9. Cellular composition and organization of the non-human primate SGZ. (A-C) Toluidine-blue stained DG semithin section (1.5 µm) showing the hilus, the SGZ and the granular cell layer. A) Panoramic view of DG, where squared areas represent different cell types. B) High magnification of type B cell. C) Microglial cell. (D-J) Ultrathin sections of the DG. (D) Panoramic view of the DG showing a hA and a microglial cell. (E) High magnification of squared area in D image, showing the large horizontal astrocytic expansion, with intermediate filaments. (F) High magnification of squared area in D, showing lisosomes of the activated microglial cell. (G) Panoramic view of the DG showing a rA and a type D cell. (H) High magnification of squared area in G image, showing astrocytic cytoplasm details pointing out its dense bodies (arrowhead). (I) High magnification of squared area in G image, showing intermediate filaments, some of them surround the nucleus. (J) Detail of type D cell presenting scarce cytoplasm and lax chromatin. Scale-bar: A=10µm; B and C=5µm; D=6µm E=µm; F=2µm; G=6µm; H=1µm ;I=600nm and J=2µm. SGZ=subgranular zone, B=type B cell, M=microglial cell, hA=horizontal astrocyte, rA=radial astrocyte and D=type D cell.

## Neural Stem Cells in Non-human Primates hippocampus

Adult neurogenesis within the SGZ of the hippocampal dentate gyrus has been most intensively studied within the brains of rodents such as mice and rats. However little is known about the cell types and the processes involved in adult neurogenesis within non-human primates.

Initial works on hippocampal neurogenesis in the rhesus monkey (Old World primates) by Eckenhoff and Rackick [79] and Kornack and Rackic [80] as well as in the common marmoset (a New World monkey) by Gould et al. [81] showed that new neurons are added to the DG of adult monkeys.

At light microscopy, toluidine blue stained semithin sections of adult marmoset hippocampus show mostly isolated astrocytes and less frequently associated to one-two type D cells. Astrocytes are clearly identified as cells with pale nuclear matrix with small chromatin clumps and light cytoplasm, which look clearly different to the adjacent granular neurons (Figure 9A). Astrocytes localize along the SGZ. While type D cells are abundant and morphologically identifiable in mice, in non-human primates type D cells are scarce and the differences with granular cell neurons is not so evident. By other hand, abundant active microglial cells characterized by dark cytoplasm and refractive lysosomes are also observed within the SGZ (Figure 9A-C).

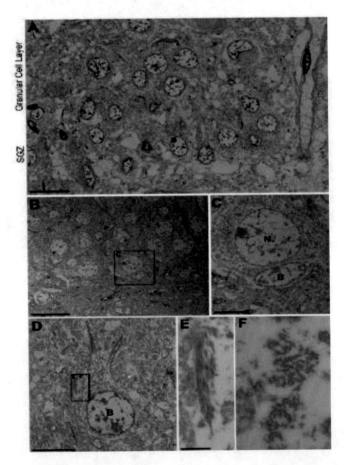

Figure 10. Cellular composition and organization of the human DG. (A) Toluidine-blue stained DG semithin section (15 µm) showing the SGZ and GCL. (B-F) Ultrathin section of the DG. (B) EM panoramic view of the SGZ. (C) High magnification of squared area in B image, showing a detail of type B cell close to a granular neuron. (D) Type B cell with cytoplasmatic expansions. Preserved intermediate filaments (E) and particulated structures or crackets (F) are squared and showed at higher magnifications. Scale-bar: A and B=10µm; C and D=5µm; E and F=300nm. N=granular neuron and B=type B cell.

At EM level, astrocytes are characterized by their irregular nuclei with dispersed chromatin and small clumps of chromatin. The cytoplasm is light containing some RER cisternae, small dictiosomes and abundant mitochondria and intermediate filaments [24, 82-84]. Occasionally, lipofucsine dark bodies are also observed. Sometimes, it is possible to identify radial and horizontal astrocytes, while radial astrocytes send long radial processes; horizontal astrocytes send large horizontal expansions (Figure 9D-I). Astrocytes also present the primary cilium described previously in mice. Occasionally, type D cells are easily identified at EM, in contrast to light microscopy where this identification is more difficult. Type D cells are characterized by being electrodense (dark) cells with irregularly shaped electrodense nuclei that contain few clumps of heterochromatin. These cells also present typical intercellular spaces. The cytoplasm is scant and contains smaller mitochondria than astrocytes, free polyribosomes, microtubules and scarce RER [82] (Figure 9G and J).

## *Neural Stem Cells in Human Hippocampus*

Eriksson and cols first described the production of newly generated cells with neuronal features in dentate gyrus of humans. In 1998 in autopsy material of patients suffering from throat carcinomas at advanced age that, as part of their treatment, received a single infusion BrdU infusion to allow staging of the tumour after its removal. Using immunofluorescence, they showed co-labeling for BrdU and an specific neuronal marker, such as NeuN, Calbindin or neuron specific enolase (NSE), demonstrating that adult neurogenesis exists in human dentate gyrus [40]. More recently, Knotch and cols. have reported a detailed analysis of neurogenesis in the human hippocampus across the lifespan from 0 to 100 years [85]. They offer a large data set of markers associated with neurogenesis (proliferation, precursor cells, maturation and differentiation), and how the expression patterns change with aging. Their data suggest that human adult hippocampal neurogenesis declines exponentially with increasing aging in a way that is consistent with that described in rodents. Currently there are no exhaustive descriptive data of human SGZ due to poor quality cell preservation, which difficult cell characterization and identification. Frequently, preparations present disintegrated tissue and undefined cellular contours at light microscopy. Astrocytes in the SGZ cannot be distinguished from the granular neurons. Moreover all the cell types present clumps of heterochromatin (Figure 10A).

At EM some type B cells can be identified at the SGZ, characterized by light cytoplasm containing intermediate filaments, which are hardly preserved, and particulated structures or crackets, which can result from intermediate filament or other structures condensation or degradation, as a consequence of fixation and preservation (Figure 10 B-E). In the dentate gyrus these intermediated filaments and crackets only appear in the SGZ astrocytes and are not observed in the granular neurons at the GCL. In human, astrocytes have not been subdivided into radial astrocytes and horizontal astrocytes. Type D cells previously described in mice and non-human primate SGZ have not yet been described in human at electron microscopy level. This could be due to the lack of cell preservation in human material and also to decrease in the number and neurogenesis in human. However, DCX+ and PSA-NCAM+ cells have been described at optical microscopy, which could correspond to type D cells [85]. The finding of neurogenesis in adult humans suggests new therapeutic strategies for replacing neurons that have been lost to brain trauma or neurodegenerative disease and may represent a mechanism of adult "neuroplasticity" previously unrecognized in humans [40].

## Conclusion

Neural stem cells have been identified as a subtype of astrocytes in the SVZ and the SGZ of adult brain from rodent to humans. Through evolution neural stem cells have preserved some characteristic ultrastructural and morphological features such as, the presence of intermediate filaments in their cytoplasm, irregular and invaginated nucleus, which often form one-two inner nuclear fusions and the presence of a single cilium, which appears in contact with the cerebrospinal fluid in the lateral ventricles in the case of the SVZ. This cilium plays an important role in the cell function, as Golgi apparatus and RER surround the base of the cilia, which is not observed in the other cell types. Interestingly, during evolution astrocytes increase the number of organelles and intermediate filaments, being more prominent in human than in non-human primates and rodent and the clumps of chromatin in the nucleus appears laxer.

## Acknowledgments

The support by Ministerio de Ciencia e Innovacion (SAF2008-01274 to M.S.S.P and J.M.G.V and AP2010-4264 to A.C.S), PROMETEO from Generalitat Valenciana (GVPROMETEO 2009-011), Red de Terapia Celular TerCel (RETICS) from Instituto de Salud Carlos III and CIBERNED is gratefully acknowledged.

## References

[1] Ramón y Cajal S. *Degeneration and regeneration of the nervous system.*: New York: Oxford University Press, American Branch, 1928.
[2] Altman J., Das G. D. Autoradiographic and histological evidence of postnatal hippocampal neurogenesis in rats. *J Comp Neurol* 1965;124:319-335.
[3] Alvarez-Buylla A., Garcia-Verdugo J. M. Neurogenesis in adult subventricular zone. *J Neurosci* 2002;22:629-634.
[4] Gage F. H. Mammalian neural stem cells. *Science* 2000;287:1433-1438.
[5] Seri B., Garcia-Verdugo J. M., McEwen B. S., Alvarez-Buylla A. Astrocytes give rise to new neurons in the adult mammalian hippocampus. *J Neurosci* 2001;21:7153-7160.
[6] Doetsch F., Caille I., Lim D. A., Garcia-Verdugo J. M., Alvarez-Buylla A. Subventricular zone astrocytes are neural stem cells in the adult mammalian brain. *Cell* 1999;97:703-716.
[7] Johansson C. B., Momma S., Clarke D. L., Risling M., Lendahl U., Frisen J. Identification of a neural stem cell in the adult mammalian central nervous system. *Cell* 1999;96:25-34.
[8] Lie D. C., Song H., Colamarino S. A, Ming G. L., Gage F. H. Neurogenesis in the adult brain: new strategies for central nervous system diseases. *Annu Rev Pharmacol Toxicol* 2004;44:399-421.
[9] Rossi F., Cattaneo E. Opinion: neural stem cell therapy for neurological diseases: dreams and reality. *Nat Rev Neurosci* 2002;3:401-409.

[10] Sauer F. Mitosis in the neural tube. *J Comp Neurol* 935;62:377-405.
[11] Kosodo Y., Roper K., Haubensak W., Marzesco A. M., Corbeil D., Huttner W. B. Asymmetric distribution of the apical plasma membrane during neurogenic divisions of mammalian neuroepithelial cells. *Embo J* 2004;23:2314-2324.
[12] Rakic P. A small step for the cell, a giant leap for mankind: a hypothesis of neocortical expansion during evolution. *Trends Neurosci* 1995;18:383-388.
[13] Haubensak W., Attardo A., Denk W., Huttner W. B. Neurons arise in the basal neuroepithelium of the early mammalian telencephalon: a major site of neurogenesis. *Proc Natl Acad Sci US A* 2004;101:3196-3201.
[14] Noctor S. C., Martinez-Cerdeno V., Ivic L., Kriegstein A. R. Cortical neurons arise in symmetric and asymmetric division zones and migrate through specific phases. *Nat Neurosci* 2004;7:136-144.
[15] Noctor S. C., Martinez-Cerdeno V., Kriegstein A. R. Contribution of intermediate progenitor cells to cortical histogenesis. *Arch Neurol* 2007;64:639-642.
[16] Boulder C. Embryonic vertebrate central nervous system: revised terminology. The Boulder Committee. *Anat Rec* 1970;166:257-261.
[17] Hinds J. W., Ruffett T. L. Cell proliferation in the neural tube: an electron microscopic and golgi analysis in the mouse cerebral vesicle. *Z Zellforsch Mikrosk Anat* 1971;115:226-264.
[18] Rakic P. Developmental and evolutionary adaptations of cortical radial glia. *Cereb Cortex* 2003;13:541-549.
[19] Bruckner G., Biesold D. Histochemistry of glycogen deposition in perinatal rat brain: importance of radial glial cells. *J Neurocytol* 1981;10:749-757.
[20] Choi B. H., Lapham L. W. Radial glia in the human fetal cerebrum: a combined Golgi, immunofluorescent and electron microscopic study. *Brain Res* 1978;148:295-311.
[21] Gadisseux J. F., Evrard P. Glial-neuronal relationship in the developing central nervous system. A histochemical-electron microscope study of radial glial cell particulate glycogen in normal and reeler mice and the human fetus. *Dev Neurosci* 1985;7:12-32.
[22] Campbell K., Gotz M. Radial glia: multi-purpose cells for vertebrate brain development. *Trends Neurosci* 2002;25:235-238.
[23] Mori T., Buffo A., Gotz M. The novel roles of glial cells revisited: the contribution of radial glia and astrocytes to neurogenesis. *Curr Top Dev Biol* 2005;69:67-99.
[24] Levitt P., Rakic P. Immunoperoxidase localization of glial fibrillary acidic protein in radial glial cells and astrocytes of the developing rhesus monkey brain. *J Comp Neurol* 1980;193:815-840.
[25] Choi B. H. Prenatal gliogenesis in the developing cerebrum of the mouse. *Glia* 1988;1:308-316.
[26] Aaku-Saraste E., Oback B., Hellwig A., Huttner W. B. Neuroepithelial cells downregulate their plasma membrane polarity prior to neural tube closure and neurogenesis. *Mech Dev* 1997;69:71-81.
[27] Stoykova A., Gotz M., Gruss P., Price J. Pax6-dependent regulation of adhesive patterning, R-cadherin expression and boundary formation in developing forebrain. *Development* 1997;124:3765-3777.
[28] Misson J. P., Takahashi T., Caviness V. S. Jr. Ontogeny of radial and other astroglial cells in murine cerebral cortex. *Glia* 1991;4:138-148.

[29] Takahashi T., Misson J. P., Caviness V. S. Jr. Glial process elongation and branching in the developing murine neocortex: a qualitative and quantitative immunohistochemical analysis. *J Comp Neurol* 1990; 302:15-28.

[30] Kriegstein A., Alvarez-Buylla A. The glial nature of embryonic and adult neural stem cells. *Annu Rev Neurosci* 2009;32:149-184.

[31] Schmechel D. E., Rakic P. A Golgi study of radial glial cells in developing monkey telencephalon: morphogenesis and transformation into astrocytes. *Anat Embryol* (Berl) 1979;156:115-152.

[32] Noctor S. C., Martinez-Cerdeno V., Kriegstein A. R. Distinct behaviors of neural stem and progenitor cells underlie cortical neurogenesis. *J Comp Neurol* 2008;508:28-44.

[33] Allen E. The cessation of mitosis in the central nervous system of the albino rat. . *J. Comp. Neurol* 1912;19:547-568.

[34] Blakemore W. F., Jolly R. D. The subependymal plate and associated ependyma in the dog. An ultrastructural study. *J Neurocytol* 1972;1:69-84.

[35] Ponti G., Aimar P., Bonfanti L. Cellular composition and cytoarchitecture of the rabbit subventricular zone and its extensions in the forebrain. *J Comp Neurol* 2006;498:491-507.

[36] Morshead C. M., Reynolds B. A., Craig C. G. et al. Neural stem cells in the adult mammalian forebrain: a relatively quiescent subpopulation of subependymal cells. *Neuron* 1994;13:1071-1082.

[37] Reynolds B. A., Weiss S. Generation of neurons and astrocytes from isolated cells of the adult mammalian central nervous system. *Science* 1992;255:1707-1710.

[38] Lewis P. D. Mitotic activity in the primate subependymal layer and the genesis of gliomas. *Nature* 1968;217:974-975.

[39] McDermott K. W., Lantos P. L. Cell proliferation in the subependymal layer of the postnatal marmoset, Callithrix jacchus. *Brain Res Dev Brain Res* 1990;57:269-277.

[40] Eriksson P. S., Perfilieva E., Bjork-Eriksson T. et al. Neurogenesis in the adult human hippocampus. *Nat Med* 1998;4:1313-1317.

[41] Kirschenbaum B., Nedergaard M., Preuss A., Barami K., Fraser R. A., Goldman S. A. In vitro neuronal production and differentiation by precursor cells derived from the adult human forebrain. *Cereb Cortex* 1994;4:576-589.

[42] Mitro A., Palkovits M. Morphology of the rat brain ventricles, ependyma, and periventricular structures. *Bibl Anat* 1981:1-110.

[43] Sanai N., Tramontin A. D., Quinones-Hinojosa A. et al. Unique astrocyte ribbon in adult human brain contains neural stem cells but lacks chain migration. Nature 2004;427:740-744.

[44] Gonzalez-Perez O., Romero-Rodriguez R., Soriano-Navarro M., Garcia-Verdugo J. M., Alvarez-Buylla A. Epidermal growth factor induces the progeny of subventricular zone type B cells to migrate and differentiate into oligodendrocytes. *Stem Cells* 2009;27:2032-2043.

[45] Menn B., Garcia-Verdugo J. M., Yaschine C., Gonzalez-Perez O., Rowitch D., Alvarez-Buylla A. Origin of oligodendrocytes in the subventricular zone of the adult brain. *J Neurosci* 2006;26:7907-7918.

[46] Garcia-Verdugo J. M., Doetsch F., Wichterle H., Lim D. A., Alvarez-Buylla A. Architecture and cell types of the adult subventricular zone: in search of the stem cells. *J Neurobiol* 1998;36:234-248.

[47] Doetsch F., Garcia-Verdugo J. M., Alvarez-Buylla A. Cellular composition and three-dimensional organization of the subventricular germinal zone in the adult mammalian brain. *J Neurosci* 1997;17:5046-5061.

[48] Doetsch F., Garcia-Verdugo J. M., Alvarez-Buylla A. Regeneration of a germinal layer in the adult mammalian brain. *Proc Natl Acad Sci USA* 1999;96:11619-11624.

[49] Tavazoie M., Van der Veken L., Silva-Vargas V. et al. A specialized vascular niche for adult neural stem cells. *Cell Stem Cell* 2008;3:279-288.

[50] Gil-Perotin S., Alvarez-Buylla A., Garcia-Verdugo J. M. Identification and characterization of neural progenitor cells in the adult mammalian brain. *Adv Anat Embryol Cell Biol* 2009;203:1-101, ix.

[51] Mercier F., Kitasako J. T., Hatton G. I. Anatomy of the brain neurogenic zones revisited: fractones and the fibroblast/macrophage network. *J Comp Neurol* 2002;451:170-188.

[52] Mercier F., Kitasako J. T., Hatton G. I. Fractones and other basal laminae in the hypothalamus. *J Comp Neurol* 2003;455:324-340.

[53] Mercier F., Schanack J., Saint Georges Chaumet M. Fractones: Home and conductor of the neural stem cell niche In: *Springer*, ed. *Adult neurogenesis*, 2011: 109-133.

[54] Voigt T. Development of glial cells in the cerebral wall of ferrets: direct tracing of their transformation from radial glia into astrocytes. *J Comp Neurol* 1989;289:74-88.

[55] Spassky N., Merkle F T., Flames N., Tramontin A. D., Garcia-Verdugo J. M., Alvarez-Buylla A. Adult ependymal cells are postmitotic and are derived from radial glial cells during embryogenesis. *J Neurosci* 2005;25:10-18.

[56] Tramontin A. D., Garcia-Verdugo J. M., Lim D. A., Alvarez-Buylla A. Postnatal development of radial glia and the ventricular zone (VZ): a continuum of the neural stem cell compartment. *Cereb Cortex* 2003;13:580-587.

[57] Merkle F. T., Alvarez-Buylla A. Neural stem cells in mammalian development. *Curr Opin Cell Biol* 2006;18:704-709.

[58] Mirzadeh Z., Merkle F T., Soriano-Navarro M., Garcia-Verdugo J. M., Alvarez-Buylla A. Neural stem cells confer unique pinwheel architecture to the ventricular surface in neurogenic regions of the adult brain. *Cell Stem Cell* 2008;3:265-278.

[59] Kornack D. R., Rakic P. The generation, migration, and differentiation of olfactory neurons in the adult primate brain. *Proc Natl Acad Sci USA* 2001;98:4752-4757.

[60] Gil-Perotin S., Duran-Moreno M., Belzunegui S., Luquin M. R., Garcia-Verdugo J. M. Ultrastructure of the subventricular zone in Macaca fascicularis and evidence of a mouse-like migratory stream. *J Comp Neurol* 2009;514:533-554.

[61] Sawamoto K., Hirota Y., Alfaro-Cervello C. et al. Cellular composition and organization of the subventricular zone and rostral migratory stream in the adult and neonatal common marmoset brain. *J Comp Neurol*; 519:690-713.

[62] Pincus D. W., Harrison-Restelli C., Barry J. et al. In vitro neurogenesis by adult human epileptic temporal neocortex. *Clin Neurosurg* 1997;44:17-25.

[63] Quinones-Hinojosa A., Sanai N., Soriano-Navarro M. et al. Cellular composition and cytoarchitecture of the adult human subventricular zone: a niche of neural stem cells. *J Comp Neurol* 2006;494:415-434.

[64] Galan L., Gomez-Pinedo U., Vela-Souto A. et al. Subventricular zone in motor neuron disease with frontotemporal dementia. *Neurosci Lett*;499:9-13.

[65] Marti-Fabregas J., Romaguera-Ros M., Gomez-Pinedo U. et al. Proliferation in the human ipsilateral subventricular zone after ischemic stroke. *Neurology*;74:357-365.

[66] Wang C., Liu F., Liu Y. Y. et al. Identification and characterization of neuroblasts in the subventricular zone and rostral migratory stream of the adult human brain. *Cell Res*;.21:1534-1550.

[67] Ge S., Goh E. L., Sailor K. A., Kitabatake Y., Ming G. L., Song H. GABA regulates synaptic integration of newly generated neurons in the adult brain. *Nature* 2006;439:589-593.

[68] Kempermann G., Jessberger S., Steiner B., Kronenberg G. Milestones of neuronal development in the adult hippocampus. *Trends Neurosci* 2004;27:447-452.

[69] Markakis E. A., Gage F. H. Adult-generated neurons in the dentate gyrus send axonal projections to field CA3 and are surrounded by synaptic vesicles. *J Comp Neurol* 1999;406:449-460.

[70] van Praag H., Schinder A. F., Christie B. R., Toni N., Palmer T. D., Gage F. H. Functional neurogenesis in the adult hippocampus. *Nature* 2002;415:1030-1034.

[71] Aimone J. B., Wiles J., Gage F. H. Potential role for adult neurogenesis in the encoding of time in new memories. *Nat Neurosci* 2006;9:723-727.

[72] Deng Y. B., Ye W. B., Hu Z. Z. et al. Intravenously administered BMSCs reduce neuronal apoptosis and promote neuronal proliferation through the release of VEGF after stroke in rats. *Neurol Res* 2010;32:148-156.

[73] Garcia A. D., Doan N. B., Imura T., Bush T. G., Sofroniew M. V. GFAP-expressing progenitors are the principal source of constitutive neurogenesis in adult mouse forebrain. *Nat Neurosci* 2004;7:1233-1241.

[74] Seri B., Garcia-Verdugo J. M., Collado-Morente L., McEwen B. S., Alvarez-Buylla A. Cell types, lineage, and architecture of the germinal zone in the adult dentate gyrus. *J Comp Neurol* 2004;478:359-378.

[75] Steiner B., Klempin F., Wang L., Kott M., Kettenmann H., Kempermann G. Type-2 cells as link between glial and neuronal lineage in adult hippocampal neurogenesis. *Glia* 2006;54:805-814.

[76] Suh H., Consiglio A., Ray J., Sawai T., D'Amour K. A., Gage F. H. In vivo fate analysis reveals the multipotent and self-renewal capacities of Sox2+ neural stem cells in the adult hippocampus. *Cell Stem Cell* 2007;1:515-528.

[77] Amador-Arjona A., Elliott J., Miller A. et al. Primary cilia regulate proliferation of amplifying progenitors in adult hippocampus: implications for learning and memory. *J Neurosci*;31:9933-9944.

[78] Breunig J. J., Sarkisian M. R., Arellano J. I. et al. Primary cilia regulate hippocampal neurogenesis by mediating sonic hedgehog signaling. *Proc Natl Acad Sci USA* 2008;105:13127-13132.

[79] Eckenhoff M. F., Rakic P. Nature and fate of proliferative cells in the hippocampal dentate gyrus during the life span of the rhesus monkey. *J Neurosci* 1988;8:2729-2747.

[80] Kornack D. R., Rakic P. Continuation of neurogenesis in the hippocampus of the adult macaque monkey. Proc Natl Acad Sci U S A 1999;96:5768-5773.
[81] Gould E., Tanapat P., McEwen B. S., Flugge G., Fuchs E. Proliferation of granule cell precursors in the dentate gyrus of adult monkeys is diminished by stress. *Proc Natl Acad Sci USA* 1998;95:3168-3171.
[82] Ngwenya L. B., Rosene D. L., Peters A. An ultrastructural characterization of the newly generated cells in the adult monkey dentate gyrus. *Hippocampus* 2008;18:210-220.
[83] Rakic P. Mode of cell migration to the superficial layers of fetal monkey neocortex. *J Comp Neurol* 1972;145:61-83.
[84] Rickmann M., Amaral D. G., Cowan W. M. Organization of radial glial cells during the development of the rat dentate gyrus. *J Comp Neurol* 1987;264:449-479.
[85] Knoth R., Singec I., Ditter M. et al. Murine features of neurogenesis in the human hippocampus across the lifespan from 0 to 100 years. *PLoS* One 2010;5:e8809.

In: Astrocytes
Editor: Oscar González-Pérez

ISBN: 978-1-62081-558-8
© 2012 Nova Science Publishers, Inc.

*Chapter VI*

# Aging, Environmental Enrichment, Object Recognition and Astrocyte Plasticity in Dentate Gyrus

*Daniel Guerreiro Diniz[1], César Augusto Raiol Foro[1], Marcia Consentino Kronka Sosthenes[1], João Bento Torres[1], Pedro Fernando da Costa Vasconcelos,[2] Cristovam Wanderley, and Picanço Diniz[1,\*]*

[1]Universidade Federal do Pará, Instituto de Ciências Biológicas,
Laboratório de Investigações em Neurodegeneração e Infecção,
Hospital Universitário João de Barros Barreto, Belém, Pará, Brazil
[2]Unit of Arbovirology and Hemorrhagic Fevers,
Evandro Chagas Institute, Belém, Pará, Brazil

## Abstract

Acquisition and retrieval of spatial information are hippocampal-dependent tasks that can be impaired by structural/functional changes induced by aging. Episodic-like and spatial memory are hippocampal-dependent tasks, as they are selectively disrupted by fornix lesions, by lesions of the dorsal and/or ventral hippocampus, by disruption of the CA3 network, or by hippocampal infusion of NMDA and AMPA receptor antagonists. In the present chapter we intend to review the available literature in murine models where object recognition was assessed and correlated with astrocyte changes in the hippocampal formation.

We correlated performed behavioral assessments with morphology and laminar distribution of astrocytes in dentate gyrus in both aged and young mice housed from weaning, either in impoverished or enriched environments.

---

[\*] Corresponding author: Cristovam Wanderley Picanço Diniz; Address: Universidade Federal do Pará, Instituto de Ciências Biológicas, Departamento de Morfologia, Laboratório de Investigações em Neurodegeneração e Infecção, Hospital Universitário João de Barros Barreto, Rua Mundurucus 4487, Guamá, CEP 66073-000 Belém, Pará, Brazil; Phone 0055 (91)32016756; Fax 0055 (91) 32016756; E-mail: cwpdiniz@gmail.com.

From our previous and present results we have learned that in the dentate gyrus the number and morphology of astrocytes change with both aging and enriched environment in a layer-dependent fashion and the impoverished condition is associated with abnormal cognitive development and an altered laminar distribution of astrocytes. A quantitative analysis of the laminar distribution of the astrocytes in the dentate gyrus revealed that the molecular layer developed astrocytosis in response to both environmental enrichment and aging, the polymorphic layer was altered only by aging and granular layer did not change de number of astrocytes.

Because aging and enriched environment induced astrocytosis in the molecular layer of the dentate gyrus, the main target of the entorhinal-to-dentate projection, we speculate that those two conditions may induce the proliferation of different astrocyte phenotypes. Paradoxically, as compared with young subjects, aged mice from enriched environment showed a higher degree of astrocytes shrinkage than age-matched subjects from impoverished environment. Taken together, our results are consistent with previous reports showing that impoverished or enriched environments could prevent or preserve respectively, normal cognitive development. We suggest that astroglial plasticity may represent at least part of the circuitry groundwork for improvements in behavioral performance in both young and aged brain.

**Keywords**: Environment, aging, episodic-like memory, spatial learning and memory, astrocytes, stereology, morphometry

## Introduction

An enriched environment for rodents has been defined as social interactions with conspecific and a stimulation of exploratory and motor behavior with a variety of toys, ladders, tunnels, rope, bridges, and running wheels for voluntary physical exercise changed periodically, whereas an impoverished environment is reduced to social interactions. Compared to those reared in impoverished environments, rodents reared in enriched environments exhibit increases in brain size and weight, neurogenesis in the dentate gyrus, number and area of synapses, dendritic branching and density, gliogenesis, and production of neurotrophic factors (Rosenzweig and Bennett, 1996, Kolb and Whishaw, 1998, Rampon and Tsien, 2000, van Praag et al., 2000). Coherently these environmental conditions affect subsequent cognitive performance (Kempermann et al., 1997, Kleim et al., 1997, Duffy et al., 2001, Teather et al., 2002)and enhances learning and memory with higher levels of marker proteins for neuronal plasticity (Mattson et al., 2001, Will et al., 2004, Nithianantharajah and Hannan, 2006).

On the other hand all species so far investigated present cognitive decline during aging, and several studies have revealed age-related increases in both microglia and astrocytes (Pilegaard and Ladefoged, 1996, Long et al., 1998, Mouton et al., 2002). Because an enriched environment improves a variety of brain functions, there has been increased interest in integrated studies combining environmental manipulation and aging (Burke and Barnes, 2006, Mora et al., 2007). For example, exposure to an enriched environment reduced the spatial memory decline in aged subjects in association with increases in neurogenesis and gliogenesis, and changes in nitric oxide, glutamate, and GABA (Eriksson et al., 1998, Soffie et al., 1999, Law et al., 2002, Frick and Fernandez, 2003, Arnaiz et al., 2004, Bennett et al.,

2006, Colas et al., 2006, Segovia et al., 2006, Harburger et al., 2007, Iso et al., 2007, Mora et al., 2007, Piedrafita et al., 2007).

Although studies regarding environmental effects on brain plasticity have focused on altered neuronal morphology, it has been demonstrated that strong morphological changes also occur in glial cells (Sirevaag and Greenough, 1987, Komitova et al., 2002). Integrated studies involving aging, environment, and glial changes are now frequent because astrocytes seem to be implicated in a number of local hippocampal regulation processes that affect learning and memory (Junjaud et al., 2006, Magistretti, 2006, Mothet et al., 2006, Todd et al., 2006, Perea and Araque, 2007).For example, it has been demonstrated that aged mice living in an enriched environment, or with running wheels, had substantially more hippocampal neurogenesis than age-matched controls, and this cellular plasticity was associated with improvements in learning parameters (Kempermann et al., 2002, van Praag et al., 2005). Paradoxically, the hippocampal astrocytes were smaller in size and number in aged rats that grew up in enriched environments compared to age-matched controls (Soffie et al., 1999). On the other hand it has been suggested that astrocytes may exhibit transient responses to the stress history of the individual rat rather than long-term adaptive responses to differential effects of rearing in complex or laboratory cage environments (Sirevaag et al., 1991). These and other data (Chadashvili and Peterson, 2006, Billard and Rouaud, 2007) demonstrate that non-neuronal plasticity associated with environment and aging is not well understood (Markham and Greenough, 2004).

Furthermore, aged and young adult mice of different strains exhibit different cognitive impairments in the performance of hippocampal-dependent tasks after a period of living in impoverished environments (Brooks et al., 2005, Murphy et al., 2006a, Harburger et al., 2007). In addition a series of recent studies in similar mouse strains demonstrated that the molecular mechanisms associated with cognitive decline during aging involve physiological processes that are not fully developed in young adult mice (Han et al., 2006, Murphy et al., 2006b, Nguyen, 2006, Droge and Schipper, 2007). Finally, within a given brain region, several types of astrocytes populations can coexist and at least nine morphological distinct types have been described (Emsley and Macklis, 2006).Each one of these types may express a variety of physiological roles (Matyash and Kettenmann, 2010) and antigens profiles (Jinno, 2011).

Thus, there are many open questions regarding how astrocytic changes associated with environmental changes and aging, impact cognitive functions and how different cellular and molecular processes possibly contribute to these processes. Since it has been previously described that astrocytes directly contribute to the long term potentiation in the entorhinal-to-dentate gyrus projection (Allen et al, 2009; Ben Menachem-Zidon et al. 2011) and LTP is essential for spatial learning and memory we previously investigated possible relationships between spatial memory decline and changes in the laminar distribution of dentate gyrus astrocytes on aged mice (Diniz et al., 2010).In particular we examined whether young adult (6 months old) and aged (20 months old) mice that grew up in large groups in either enriched or impoverished environments could form integrated memories of the spatio-temporal context in which objects were presented. We also assessed changes in spatial memory with a long-term learning procedure in a water maze paradigm (Morris, 1984) in a different set of subjects (young adult and aged) that lived in impoverished or enriched environments.

In the present chapter we integrated previous analysis of the astrocytes laminar distribution and behavior (Diniz et al., 2010) with three dimensional analyses of the morphological features of astrocytes. To do so, we selected astrocytes from DG-molecular layer where synaptic potentiation at the entorhinal-to-dentate granular projection is dependent of glutamate exocytosis from astrocytes (Jourdain et al., 2007).

## Learning and Memory Changes

We have learned from our previous results (Diniz et al., 2010) that only young adult and aged mice from the enriched environment were able to integrate object recognition in a spatio-temporal context. The subjects from impoverished environments were unable to make the appropriate distinctions (Figure 1). In the spatial memory component of episodic-like memory (Where?) young and aged subjects housed in enriched conditions spent respectively significantly more time in the displaced than stationary objects (two-tail t-test, $p<0.05$). In the identity and temporal memory components (What? and When?) young and aged subjects housed in enriched conditions spent respectively significantly more time in the old than recent objects (two-tail t-test, $p<0.05$).

From water maze tests it became clear that environment and aging affect the ability of an animal to learn and remember the position of a hidden platform. As previously demonstrated (Diniz et al., 2010) the IY, EY, and EA groups were able to learn and remember the position of the hidden platform, but the IA group did not learn the position of the platform. Figure 2 represents individual absolute values (circles) and the average of daily distance (m) for each group (squares). Note that, related to the $1^{st}$ day, IY and EY reduced significantly travelled distance on the $3^{rd}$ day whereas EA and IA only in the $5^{th}$ and $7^{th}$ days respectively. The tracking of the swimming trajectories at the $5^{th}$ day in Figure 2 bottomrevealed that an enriched environment improved the ability to devise a strategy for reaching the hidden platform in both young and aged groups. ANOVA two-way applied to the learning rate revealed that age and environment ($P <0.05$) affected the performances in the Water-maze with no interaction between those variables.

## Astrocytes Morphometrical and Stereological Changes

Figure 3 shows a series of photomicrographs of DG - molecular layer astrocytes and the equivalent three-dimensional reconstructions (top left) from Diniz et al., unpublished results. Pictures were taken every 1μm through the z-axis of each section from a representative astrocyte of each experimental group. In 3-D reconstructions different colors distinguish the order of the segments and cell bodies. We have selected to illustrate typical astrocytes with morphometric features closer to the mean group values.

Figures 4 and 5 illustrate respectively equivalent dendrograms for three-dimensional reconstructions of the same astrocytes previously shown in Figure 3, and quantitative aspects of the morphometrical analysis of each experimental group (Diniz et al unpublished results). Note that aged mice from both impoverished and enriched groups as compared to young ones showed a significant degree of shrinkage on its branches.

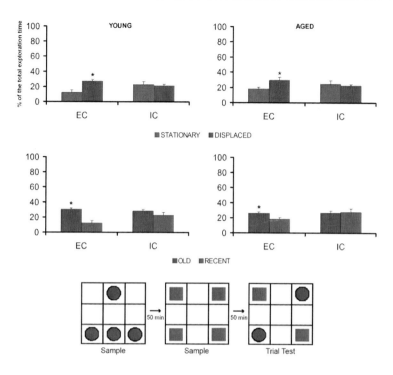

Figure 1. Episodic-like memory tests. Diagram of the experimental designs and results for object recognition integrated tests (Episodic-like memory), based on (Dere et al., 2007). Values on the Y-axes represent the time of exploration for each object as a percentage of the total time of exploration. Labels on the X-axes indicate experimental groups. Bars indicate average values ± S.E.M for the indicated groups. Red and green color filled bars represent differences between objects (displaced vs stationary, old vs recent,,). (*) = two-tail t-test; $p<0.05$). IA = impoverished aged; EA = enriched aged; IY = impoverished young; EY = enriched young. Adapted from (Diniz et al., 2010).

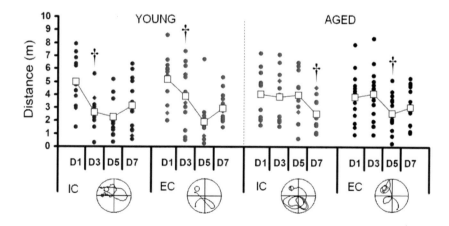

Figure 2. Water maze test. Top: Individual absolute values (circles) and the average of daily distance (squares) for each group. As compared to the 1st day, IY and EY reduced significantly travelled distance on the 3rd day; whereas EA and IA only in the 5th and days respectively. Bottom: Tracking of the swimming trajectories at the 5th day. Note that an enriched environment improved the ability to reach the hidden platform in both young and aged groups.(†) = significant reduction in escape latency as compared with 1st day test (one-way ANOVA $p<0.05$).IA = impoverished aged; EA = enriched aged; IY = impoverished young; EY = enriched young. Adapted from (Diniz et al., 2010).

Paradoxically aged mice from enriched environment present a higher degree of shrinkage than the ones from impoverished environment (Figure 4) and a significant reduction in the number of branching points (Figure 5 A). Indeed the aging process associated with impoverished environment revealed astrocytes with smaller length, area and volume of segments (Figure 5 D, F and H) as compared to the astrocytes of equivalent young group, whereas the ones from the subjects raised in enriched environment had all morphometric variables reduced significantly (Figure 5 A-H).

Figure 6 illustrates in medium power a series of pictures from GFAP-immunolabeled sections of equivalent regions of the dentate gyrus molecular layer of EY, EA, IY and IA. Note that astrocytes from young mice (EY and IY) are larger, thicker and less numerous than the ones from aged mice (EA and IA) and these differences seem to be more conspicuous between EY and EA than IY and IA.

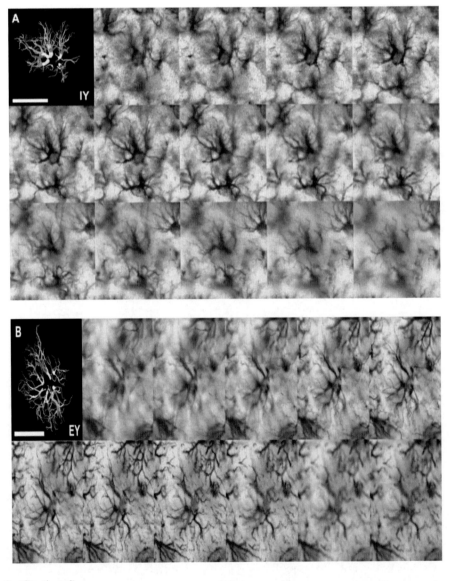

Figure 3. (Continued).

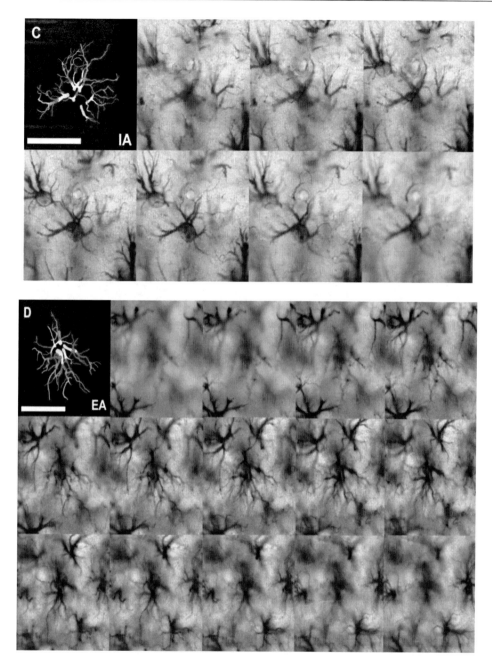

Figure 3. Serial phtomicrographics of DG - molecular layer astrocytes and the equivalent three dimensional reconstruction. Pictures were taken from a representative astrocyte of each experimental group, every 1μm through the depth section. We have chosen astrocytes with morphometric features closer to the group mean values. Striking differences were detected in the three-dimensional reconstructions between the aged and young adult groups. Less marked difference was found between impoverished and enriched environment groups. IA = impoverished aged; EA = enriched aged; IY = impoverished young; EY = enriched young.

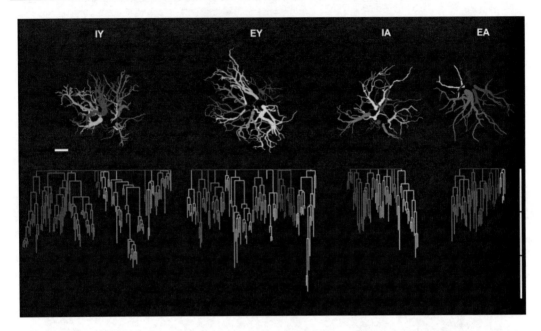

Figure 4. Top: representative 3-dimensionally reconstructed DG-molecular layer astrocytes of the young (EY, IY) and aged (EA, IA) mice. Astrocytes selected were representatives of the molecular layer of the dentate gyrus. Bottom: linear dendrogram of each astrocyte arbor with the length of each branch segment is displayed to scale as vertical lines and sister branches is horizontally displaced. Dendrogram was plotted and analyzed with Neuroexplorer (MicroBrightField). Branches of the same parental (primary branch) trunk are shown in one color. As compared to young, aged mice show significant shrinkage of astrocytes branches. Scale bar = 75μm.

Figure 7 gives graphic representations of the total numbers of astrocytes in the molecular layer of the dentate gyrus and behavioral performances on episodic-like memory tests. On average, aged mice from the enriched environment exhibited higher numbers of astrocytes in the molecular layer than young mice housed in a similar environment. Aging and enriched environment seem to promote an additive hyperplasia of astrocytes in this layer. Indeed the estimations of the astrocytes number in the molecular layer of dentate gyrus revealed significant differences induced by age and environmental changes (two-way ANOVA, $p<0.05$), but no interactions among these variables.

In all cases, the variance introduced by methodological procedures was less than 50% of the observed group variance, giving a ratio of $CE^2/CV^2 < 0.5$ (Slomianka and West, 2005). The biological variation represented 77 – 99.6% of the total variation. Figure 7 also illustrates average behavioral performances in the episodic-like memory test (right Y-axis and gray horizontal rectangles).

We defined as 70% the minimal acceptable difference in the time of exploration between the objects to indicate that the object recognition had occurred. The dotted line in the figure points to this level, indicating that on average IA subjects did not reach the criteria. Note that the average values of discrimination index reproduced in the selected subjects for counting reveals the same tendencies observed in the water maze and episodic-like memory tests. However, we did not find a simple correlation between the astrocytes numbers and episodic-like memory performances.

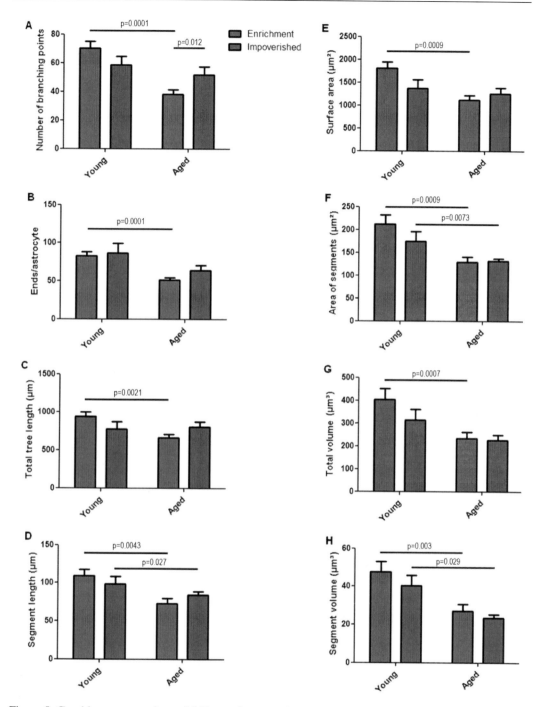

Figure 5. Graphic representations of 3-D morphometry. Note that aging is associated with significant shrinkage. Segment analysis demonstrated that an impoverished environment reduces length, area and volumes of segments (D, F and H) whereas aged mice raised in an enriched environment showed a reduction in the mean values of all variables (A-H). As compared with impoverished environment, the number of branching points were more affected by aging in the subjects from enriched environment (A). p values after two-tail t-tests are indicated.

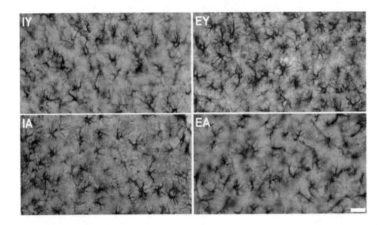

Figure 6. Astrocytes from molecular layer of mice dentate gyrus. A series of pictures fromGFAPimmunolabeled sections to illustrate distribution and morphology of astrocytes. Pictures were taken from equivalent regions of the dentate gyrus molecular layer of EY, EA, IY and IA. Note that astrocytes from young mice (EY and IY) are larger, thicker and less numerous than the ones from aged mice (EA and IA) and these differences seem to be more conspicuous between EY and EA than between IY and IA. IA = impoverished environment, aged mice; EA = enriched environment, aged mice; IY = impoverished environment, young mice; EY = enriched environment, young mice.

Taken together the results demonstrate that a 24-h per day complex environmental enrichment had differential effects on the number of astrocytes in the dentate gyrus and on the performances in episodic-like and water maze memory tests among young and aged female albino Swiss mice. After 20 months, mice reared under impoverished conditions exhibited cognitive dysfunctions in both tests. After 6 months, mice reared under the same conditions also exhibited changes in the performances in episodic-like memory and water maze tests. In contrast, continuous environmental enrichment, beginning early in life (21$^{st}$ postnatal day), induced astrocyte hyperplasia in the molecular layer, preserved episodic-like memory, and reduced the impact of aging on the Morris water maze spatial memory.

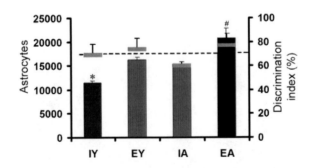

Figure 7. Graphic representation of the average values of episodic memory-like test (right Y-axis) and number of astrocytes in the molecular layer of dentate gyrus (left Y-axis) of five subjects of each experimental group. Points above 70% (dotted line) indicate the experimental group that completed the object recognition task. Note that there is not any simple correlation between the number of astrocytes and behavioral performances. IA = impoverished environment, aged mice; EA = enriched environment, aged mice; IY = impoverished environment, young mice; EY = enriched environment, young mice. (*) = IY shows less astrocytes than all other groups. (#) = EA shows more astrocytes than all other groups (two-way-ANOVA $p<0.05$). Adapted from (Diniz et al., 2010).

In addition our preliminary results of morphometric analysis (Diniz et al., unpublished results) revealed that aged mice from both impoverished and enriched groups as compared to young ones showed a significant degree of shrinkage on its branches. Taken together the results suggested that different degrees of laminar astrocytosis and morphological changes were induced in the murine dentate gyrus by environmental and aging conditions. It also suggests that an enriched environment may protect against abnormal cognitive development and cognitive decline due to aging. Because aged subjects raised in enriched conditions had improved memories compared to those raised in impoverished conditions, we speculate that the astrocytosis detected in these conditions may arise from different astrocytic phenotypes.

## Environmental Impoverishment and Aging Impacts on Morris Water-maze Performance and Episodic-like Memory

Acquisition and retrieval of spatial information are hippocampal-dependent tasks that can be impaired by structural/functional changes induced by aging (Riedel et al., 1999, D'Hooge and De Deyn, 2001, Da Silva Costa et al., 2009). Spatial memory decline has been associated with age-related changes in the brain regions involved with spatial learning, e.g., the hippocampal formation (Teather et al., 2002, Frick and Fernandez, 2003, Rosenzweig and Barnes, 2003, Wimmer et al., 2011). In the present report, the water maze tests at the $5^{th}$ day test revealed that IA subjects did not exhibit an ability to learn and remember the position of a hidden platform; in contrast IY, EY, and EA individuals did exhibit these abilities at this time windows, albeit to different extents. We did not find any significant differences in swimming speeds between young and aged mice in either the IC or the EC groups; this suggested that cognitive decline, rather than physical differences, was more likely to explain the differences in performance in the water maze task.

It has previously been confirmed that episodic-like memory in rats and mice is a hippocampal-dependent task, as it is selectively disrupted by fornix lesions, by lesions of the dorsal and/or ventral hippocampus, by disruption of the CA3 network, or by hippocampal infusion of NMDA and AMPA receptor antagonists (Daumas et al., 2004, Eacott and Norman, 2004, Ergorul and Eichenbaum, 2004, Bast et al., 2005, Li and Chao, 2008). We detected episodic-like memory impairments in both young adult and aged mice raised in impoverished conditions; thus, we reasoned that the dentate gyrus could be an important target for the pathophysiological changes associated with impoverished conditions in female albino Swiss mice. Each hippocampal region contains a distinct population of neurons that express unique molecular profiles (Zhao et al., 2001), and the dentate gyrus seems to be particularly sensitive to age-related changes (Small et al., 2004). Therefore, we speculate that spatial memory deficits in young adult mice may have different pathophysiological mechanisms than those in aged mice, and that both are additive to the influences of an impoverished environment. Indeed, when young adult and aged mice raised in IC were tested for spatial memory and learning with the water maze paradigm, the young adults were able to learn and remember the position of the hidden platform after 5 training days, but the aged mice were unable to complete the test at this time point. These results suggested that, after 6 months of impoverished conditions, the hippocampal requirements for spatial learning in young mice could be reactivated with training. As expected, memory capabilities became worse when advanced age was combined with an impoverished environment; under these conditions, learning and memory at Morris water maze took 7 days to become significant but all types of episodic-like memories deteriorated. In contrast, aged mice that grew up in enriched environments exhibited relatively unimpaired learning and memory in all memory tests. This suggested that the consolidation and retrieval mechanisms for these memories were spared under enriched environmental conditions.

## Dentate Gyrus Astrocytes, Environment, Aging, and Cognitive Decline

The pathophysiological bases for memory impairments have not yet been completely elucidated but the impact of enriched environment on glial cells has been previously described (Altman and Das, 1964). In that light, it is interesting to discuss possible connections between the quantitative astrocytic response and the cognitive protection observed with environmental enrichment. Our stereological analysis of hippocampal sections from IC aged mice revealed hyperplasia of astrocytes compared to equivalent sections from IC young adults. These differences were associated with a striking cognitive decline in IC aged mice. In contrast, EC aged mice exhibited a higher number of astrocytes in the molecular layer compared to IC aged mice. Interestingly, EA subjects exhibited the ability to form integrated memories in the spatio-temporal contexto and learned to find and remember the position of the hidden platform in the water maze test. Accordingly, the analysis of the water maze test revealed that there was a gradient between the EY (who exhibited the best learning rate) and IA (who exhibited no learning) mice. This was evidenced by the intermediate performances of IY and EA individuals. However, the molecular layer of the dentate gyrus was additively affected by both environment and aging; thus, we speculate that astrocytosis induced by environmental enrichment may have a different functional role than that induced by aging. Paradoxically our preliminary results of morphometric analysis in the molecular layer of dentate gyrus confirmed previous suggestions in the hippocampus of old rats (Soffie et al., 1999)that astrocytes from the hippocampus of enriched environment subjects as compared to the ones from impoverished environment are smaller. Taken together the results suggest that compare to young subjects of equivalent environments, aged mice from enriched conditions present more and smaller astrocytes than aged mice raised in impoverished conditions.It remains to be investigated possible implications of these differences in astrocytes. However more recently, emerging evidence indicates that the number of cells expressing biomarkers of cellular senescence increases in tissues with aging and that astrocytes in the aging brain expresses characteristics of senescence-associated secretory phenotype (Salminen et al., 2011).

One possible question to be answered is how these changes would affect astrocytic glutamate exocytosis at the entorhinal-to-dentate granular cells (perforant pathway). By this mechanism astrocytes participate in synaptic tuning in circuits involved in cognitive processing and the control of the mossy fiber-to-CA3 synaptic input (Jourdain et al., 2007). Conversely, even in the absence of neurological disease a more reactive phenotype of astrocyte is expressed during aging as part of an increased and maintained pro-inflammatory profile that may be associated with cognitive dysfunction (Godbout and Johnson, 2009). Indeed it has been demonstrated that aged astrocytes but not microglia or neurons increase the expression of TNFα, IL-1β and IL-6 in the rat brain (Campuzano et al., 2009). In addition a decrease in the ability of aged rats to sustain long-term potentiation (LTP) in the perforant pathway of the dentate gyrus was also associated with microglial activation (Lynch, 2010).We suggest that as compared with aged subjects housed in enriched conditions, the subjects raised in impoverished conditions may have an increase in the number of astrocytes with senescence-associated secretory phenotype (Lynch, 2010).

The notion that aging and impoverished environments may cause similar cellular and molecular alterations in the hippocampus is supported by another study that showed two nutritional supplements, CDP-choline and uridine monophosphate (UMP), prevented spatial memory impairments in both young IE and aged Sprague-Dawley rats (Teather and Wurtman, 2005, 2006). In the present report we have detected differential effects of impoverished environments on the memories of young adult and aged mice; a future extension of this study could be to establish quantitative correlations between pathophysiological features and behavioral performances in longitudinal studies. This would allow better resolution of the mechanisms of cognitive decline and brain plasticity related to aging.

# Conclusion

Our previous stereological and present morphometrical analysis of astrocytes revealed significant morphological changes and altered distribution of astrocytes in dentate gyrus in response to environmental conditions and aging in adult female albino Swiss mice. The presence of astroglial plasticity associated with learning and memory changes in these animals may be part of the circuitry groundwork for improvements in hippocampal-dependent behavioral performance in both young and aged brain.

# Acknowledgments

This project was sponsored by Brazilian Government research funds from CNPq to CWPD and FINEP to the Instituto Brasileiro de Neurociências (IBNnet).

# References

Altman J., Das G. D. (Autoradiographic Examination of the Effects of Enriched Environment on the Rate of Glial Multiplication in the Adult Rat Brain. *Nature* 204:1161-1163.1964).

Arnaiz S. L., D'Amico G., Paglia N., Arismendi M., Basso N., del Rosario Lores Arnaiz M. (Enriched environment, nitric oxide production and synaptic plasticity prevent the aging-dependent impairment of spatial cognition. *Mol Aspects Med* 25:91-101.2004).

Bast T., da Silva B. M., Morris R. G. (Distinct contributions of hippocampal NMDA and AMPA receptors to encoding and retrieval of one-trial place memory. *J Neurosci* 25:5845-5856.2005).

Bennett J. C., McRae P. A., Levy L. J., Frick K. M. (Long-term continuous, but not daily, environmental enrichment reduces spatial memory decline in aged male mice. *Neurobiol Learn Mem* 85:139-152.2006).

Billard J. M., Rouaud E. (Deficit of NMDA receptor activation in CA1 hippocampal area of aged rats is rescued by D-cycloserine. *Eur J Neurosci* 25:2260-2268.2007).

Brooks S. P., Pask T., Jones L., Dunnett S. B. (Behavioural profiles of inbred mouse strains used as transgenic backgrounds. II: cognitive tests. *Genes Brain Behav* 4:307-317.2005).

Burke S. N., Barnes C. A. (Neural plasticity in the ageing brain. *Nat Rev Neurosci* 7:30-40.2006).

Campuzano O., Castillo-Ruiz M. M., Acarin L., Castellano B., Gonzalez B. (Increased levels of proinflammatory cytokines in the aged rat brain attenuate injury-induced cytokine response after excitotoxic damage. *Journal of neuroscience research* 87:2484-2497.2009).

Colas D., Gharib A., Bezin L., Morales A., Guidon G., Cespuglio R., Sarda N. (Regional age-related changes in neuronal nitric oxide synthase (nNOS), messenger RNA levels and activity in SAMP8 brain. *BMC Neurosci* 7:81.2006).

Chadashvili T., Peterson D. A. (Cytoarchitecture of fibroblast growth factor receptor 2 (FGFR-2) immunoreactivity in astrocytes of neurogenic and non-neurogenic regions of the young adult and aged rat brain. *J Comp Neurol* 498:1-15.2006).

D'Hooge R., De Deyn P. P. (Applications of the Morris water maze in the study of learning and memory. *Brain Res Brain Res Rev* 36:60-90.2001).

Da Silva Costa V., Duchatelle P., Boulouard M., Dauphin F. (Selective 5-HT6 receptor blockade improves spatial recognition memory and reverses age-related deficits in spatial recognition memory in the mouse. *Neuropsychopharmacology* 34:488-500.2009).

Daumas S., Halley H., Lassalle J. M. (Disruption of hippocampal CA3 network: effects on episodic-like memory processing in C57BL/6J mice. *Eur J Neurosci* 20:597-600.2004).

Diniz D. G., Foro C. A., Rego C. M., Gloria D. A., de Oliveira F. R., Paes J. M., de Sousa A. A., Tokuhashi T. P., Trindade L. S., Turiel M. C., Vasconcelos E. G., Torres J. B., Cunnigham C., Perry V. H., Vasconcelos P. F., Diniz C. W. (Environmental impoverishment and aging alter object recognition, spatial learning, and dentate gyrus astrocytes. *Eur J Neurosci* 32:509-519.2010).

Droge W., Schipper H. M. (Oxidative stress and aberrant signaling in aging and cognitive decline. *Aging Cell* 6:361-370.2007).

Duffy S. N., Craddock K. J., Abel T., Nguyen P. V. (Environmental enrichment modifies the PKA-dependence of hippocampal LTP and improves hippocampus-dependent memory. *Learn Mem* 8:26-34.2001).

Eacott M. J., Norman G. (Integrated memory for object, place, and context in rats: a possible model of episodic-like memory? *J Neurosci* 24:1948-1953.2004).

Emsley J. G., Macklis J. D. (Astroglial heterogeneity closely reflects the neuronal-defined anatomy of the adult murine CNS. *Neuron Glia Biol* 2:175-186.2006).

Ergorul C., Eichenbaum H. (The hippocampus and memory for "what," "where," and "when". *Learn Mem* 11:397-405.2004).

Eriksson P. S., Perfilieva E., Bjork-Eriksson T., Alborn A. M., Nordborg C., Peterson D. A., Gage F. H. (Neurogenesis in the adult human hippocampus. *Nat Med* 4:1313-1317.1998).

Frick K. M., Fernandez S. M. (Enrichment enhances spatial memory and increases synaptophysin levels in aged female mice. *Neurobiol Aging* 24:615-626.2003).

Godbout J. P., Johnson R. W. (Age and Neuroinflammation: A Lifetime of Psychoneuroimmune Consequences. *Immunology and Allergy Clinics of North America* 29:321-337.2009).

Han M., Schottler F., Lei D., Dong E. Y., Bryan A., Bao J. (Bcl-2 over-expression fails to prevent age-related loss of calretinin positive neurons in the mouse dentate gyrus. *Mol Neurodegener* 1:9.2006).

Harburger L. L., Nzerem C. K., Frick K. M. (Single enrichment variables differentially reduce age-related memory decline in female mice. *Behav Neurosci* 121:679-688.2007).

Iso H., Simoda S., Matsuyama T. (Environmental change during postnatal development alters behaviour, cognitions and neurogenesis of mice. *Behav Brain Res* 179:90-98.2007).

Jinno S. (Regional and laminar differences in antigen profiles and spatial distributions of astrocytes in the mouse hippocampus, with reference to aging. *Neuroscience* 180:41-52.2011).

Jourdain P., Bergersen L. H., Bhaukaurally K., Bezzi P., Santello M., Domercq M., Matute C., Tonello F., Gundersen V., Volterra A. (Glutamate exocytosis from astrocytes controls synaptic strength. *Nature neuroscience* 10:331-339.2007).

Junjaud G., Rouaud E., Turpin F., Mothet J. P., Billard J. M. (Age-related effects of the neuromodulator D-serine on neurotransmission and synaptic potentiation in the CA1 hippocampal area of the rat. *Journal of neurochemistry* 98:1159-1166.2006).

Kempermann G., Gast D., Gage F. H. (Neuroplasticity in old age: sustained fivefold induction of hippocampal neurogenesis by long-term environmental enrichment. *Ann Neurol* 52:135-143.2002).

Kempermann G., Kuhn H. G., Gage F. H. (More hippocampal neurons in adult mice living in an enriched environment. *Nature* 386:493-495.1997).

Kleim J. A., Vij K., Ballard D. H., Greenough W. T. (Learning-dependent synaptic modifications in the cerebellar cortex of the adult rat persist for at least four weeks. *J Neurosci* 17:717-721.1997).

Kolb B., Whishaw I. Q. (Brain plasticity and behavior. *Annu Rev Psychol* 49:43-64.1998).

Komitova M., Perfilieva E., Mattsson B., Eriksson P. S., Johansson B. B. (Effects of cortical ischemia and postischemic environmental enrichment on hippocampal cell genesis and differentiation in the adult rat. *J Cereb Blood Flow Metab* 22:852-860.2002).

Law A., O' Donnell J., Gauthier S., Quirion R. (Neuronal and inducible nitric oxide synthase expressions and activities in the hippocampi and cortices of young adult, aged cognitively unimpaired, and impaired Long-Evans rats. *Neuroscience* 112:267-275.2002).

Li J. S., Chao Y. S. (Electrolytic lesions of dorsal CA3 impair episodic-like memory in rats. *Neurobiol Learn Mem* 89:192-198.2008).

Long J. M., Kalehua A. N., Muth N. J., Calhoun M. E., Jucker M., Hengemihle J. M., Ingram D. K., Mouton P. R. (Stereological analysis of astrocyte and microglia in aging mouse hippocampus. *Neurobiol Aging* 19:497-503.1998).

Lynch M. A. (Age-related neuroinflammatory changes negatively impact on neuronal function. *Frontiers in aging neuroscience* 1:6.2010).

Magistretti P. J. (Neuron-glia metabolic coupling and plasticity. *The Journal of experimental biology* 209:2304-2311.2006).

Markham J. A., Greenough W. T. (Experience-driven brain plasticity: beyond the synapse. *Neuron Glia Biol* 1:351-363.2004).

Mattson M. P., Duan W., Lee J., Guo Z. (Supression of brain aging and neurodegenerative disorders by dietary restriction and environmental enrichment: molecular mechanisms. *Mechanisms of Ageing and Development* 122:757-778.2001).

Matyash V., Kettenmann H. (Heterogeneity in astrocyte morphology and physiology. *Brain research reviews* 63:2-10.2010).

Mora F., Segovia G., Del Arco A. (Aging, plasticity and environmental enrichment: Structural changes and neurotransmitter dynamics in several areas of the brain. *Brain Res Rev* 55:78-88.2007).

Morris R. (Developments of a water-maze procedure for studying spatial learning in the rat. *J Neurosci Methods* 11:47-60.1984).

Mothet J. P., Rouaud E., Sinet P. M., Potier B., Jouvenceau A., Dutar P., Videau C., Epelbaum J., Billard J. M. (A critical role for the glial-derived neuromodulator D-serine in the age-related deficits of cellular mechanisms of learning and memory. *Aging Cell* 5:267-274.2006).

Mouton P. R., Long J. M., Lei D. L., Howard V., Jucker M., Calhoun M. E., Ingram D. K. (Age and gender effects on microglia and astrocyte numbers in brains of mice. *Brain Res* 956:30-35.2002).

Murphy G. G., Rahnama N. P., Silva A. J. (Investigation of age-related cognitive decline using mice as a model system: behavioral correlates. *Am J Geriatr Psychiatry* 14:1004-1011.2006a).

Murphy G. G., Shah V., Hell J. W., Silva A. J. (Investigation of age-related cognitive decline using mice as a model system: neurophysiological correlates. *Am J Geriatr Psychiatry* 14:1012-1021.2006b).

Nguyen P. V. (Comparative plasticity of brain synapses in inbred mouse strains. *J Exp Biol* 209:2293-2303.2006).

Nithianantharajah J., Hannan A. J. (Enriched environments, experience-dependent plasticity and disorders of the nervous system. Nature reviews 7:697-709.2006).

Perea G., Araque A. (Astrocytes potentiate transmitter release at single hippocampal synapses. *Science* 317:1083-1086.2007).

Piedrafita B., Cauli O., Montoliu C., Felipo V. (The function of the glutamate-nitric oxide-cGMP pathway in brain in vivo and learning ability decrease in parallel in mature compared with young rats. *Learn Mem* 14:254-258.2007).

Pilegaard K., Ladefoged O. (Total number of astrocytes in the molecular layer of the dentate gyrus of rats at different ages. *Anal Quant Cytol Histol* 18:279-285.1996).

Rampon C., Tsien J. Z. (Genetic analysis of learning behavior-induced structural plasticity. *Hippocampus* 10:605-609.2000).

Riedel G., Micheau J., Lam A. G., Roloff E. L., Martin S. J., Bridge H., de Hoz L., Poeschel B., McCulloch J., Morris R. G. (Reversible neural inactivation reveals hippocampal participation in several memory processes. *Nature neuroscience* 2:898-905.1999).

Rosenzweig E. S., Barnes C. A. (Impact of aging on hippocampal function: plasticity, network dynamics, and cognition. *Prog Neurobiol* 69:143-179.2003).

Rosenzweig M. R., Bennett E. L. (Psychobiology of plasticity: effects of training and experience on brain and behavior. *Behav Brain Res* 78:57-65.1996).

Salminen A., Ojala J., Kaarniranta K., Haapasalo A., Hiltunen M., Soininen H. (Astrocytes in the aging brain express characteristics of senescence-associated secretory phenotype. *Eur J Neurosci* 34:3-11.2011).

Segovia G., Yague A. G., Garcia-Verdugo J. M., Mora F. Environmental enrichment promotes neurogenesis and changes the extracellular concentrations of glutamate and GABA in the hippocampus of aged rats. *Brain Res Bull* 70:8-14.2006.

Sirevaag A. M., Black J. E., Greenough W. T. (Astrocyte hypertrophy in the dentate gyrus of young male rats reflects variation of individual stress rather than group environmental complexity manipulations. *Exp Neurol* 111:74-79.1991).

Sirevaag A. M., Greenough W. T. (Differential rearing effects on rat visual cortex synapses. III. Neuronal and glial nuclei, boutons, dendrites, and capillaries. *Brain Res* 424:320-332.1987).

Slomianka L., West M. Estimators of the precision of stereological estimates: an example based on the CA1 pyramidal cell layer of rats. *Neuroscience* 136:757–767.2005.

Small S. A., Chawla M. K., Buonocore M., Rapp P. R., Barnes C. A. (Imaging correlates of brain function in monkeys and rats isolates a hippocampal subregion differentially vulnerable to aging. *Proc Natl Acad Sci USA* 101:7181-7186.2004).

Soffie M., Hahn K., Terao E., Eclancher F. (Behavioural and glial changes in old rats following environmental enrichment. *Behav Brain Res* 101:37-49.1999).

Teather L. A., Magnusson J. E., Chow C. M., Wurtman R. J. (Environmental conditions influence hippocampus-dependent behaviours and brain levels of amyloid precursor protein in rats. *Eur J Neurosci* 16:2405-2415.2002).

Teather L. A., Wurtman R. J. (Dietary CDP-choline supplementation prevents memory impairment caused by impoverished environmental conditions in rats. *Learn Mem* 12:39-43.2005).

Teather L. A., Wurtman R. J. (Chronic administration of UMP ameliorates the impairment of hippocampal-dependent memory in impoverished rats. *J Nutr* 136:2834-2837.2006).

Todd K. J., Serrano A., Lacaille J. C., Robitaille R. (Glial cells in synaptic plasticity. *J Physiol Paris* 99:75-83.2006).

van Praag H., Kempermann G., Gage F. H. (Neural consequences of environmental enrichment. *Nature reviews* 1:191-198.2000).

van Praag H., Shubert T., Zhao C., Gage F. H. (Exercise enhances learning and hippocampal neurogenesis in aged mice. *J Neurosci* 25:8680-8685.2005).

Will B., Galani R., Kelche C., Rosenzweig M. R. (Recovery from brain injury in animals: relative efficacy of environmental enrichment, physical exercise or formal training (1990-2002). *Prog Neurobiol* 72:167-182.2004).

Wimmer M. E., Hernandez P. J., Blackwell J., Abel T. Aging impairs hippocampus-dependent long-term memory for object location in mice. *Neurobiol Aging*. 2011.

Zhao X., Lein E. S., He A., Smith S. C., Aston C., Gage F. H. (Transcriptional profiling reveals strict boundaries between hippocampal subregions. *J Comp Neurol* 441:187-196.2001).

In: Astrocytes
Editor: Oscar González-Pérez

ISBN: 978-1-62081-558-8
© 2012 Nova Science Publishers, Inc.

*Chapter VII*

# Role of Astrocytes in Viral Infections

*Cecilia Bender[1,*], Jesica Frik[2,*], and Ricardo M. Gómez[2,#]*
[1]Graduate School for Life and Health Sciences, University of Verona, Italy
[2]Biotechnology and Molecular Biology Institute,
CONICET-UNLP, La Plata, Argentina

## Abstract

Viral encephalitis is most commonly caused by neurotropic herpesviruses, enteroviruses, arboviruses, paramyxoviruses, rhabdoviruses and retroviruses. Astrocytes are a major cell population of the central nervous system (CNS) and play multiple roles in CNS development, function and responses to injury. Reactive astrocytes or astrogliosis is prominent in most CNS infections. Together with activated microglia, they play major roles in inflammatory and immune responses during viral infection. Activated astrocytes express toll-like receptors crucial for the induction of innate immune responses, including the secretion of chemokines or cytokines in response to virus agents. Astrocytes also express class II major histocompatibility complex antigens, but its role as an antigen-presenting cell is still controversial. Both protective and detrimental roles have been assigned to astrogliosis during viral infections. This chapter will summarize the role of astrocytes in CNS viral infections.

## Introduction

Several viruses have adopted different strategies to successfully bypass the blood brain barrier (BBB) and enter into the central nervous system (CNS) cells to cause several inflammatory diseases such as meningitis, encephalitis or meningoencephalitis. The symptoms may vary and most of these neurotropic viruses may either produce severe damages, remain latent

---

[*] Both authors contributed equally.
[#] Corresponding author: Ricardo M. Gómez, Instituto de Biotecnología y Biología Molecular, CCT-La Plata, CONICET- UNLP, Calle 49 y 115, 1900 La Plata, Argentina; Tel: (+54) 0221-422-6977; Fax: (+54) 0221-422-4967; E-mail: rmg@biol.unlp.edu.ar.

for long periods, or they can be reactivated to cause severe brain pathologies. Several viruses are capable to infect astrocytes, the most abundant CNS cell type. Since astrocytes play a crucial role in many normal CNS functions, infection of these cells may compromise such functions leading to serious CNS damages and neurological complications. Together with microglia, astrocytes have been involved to participate in both the innate and adaptive immune response to viral infectious agents. Reactive astrocytes can express many pattern recognition molecules as toll-like receptors and secret chemokines and cytokines. Moreover, although their role as antigen-presenting cells is still under discussion, reactive astrocytes may also express class II and class I major histocompatibility complex antigens as well as B-7 and B-40 co-stimulatory molecules. In the present chapter, we will discuss the role of astrocytes during CNS viral infection, focusing on their ability to exert both an innate or adaptive immune response. The protective and detrimental role assigned to astrocyte activation process during viral infections is another conflicting aspect that will be examined in this chapter.

## Viral Infections of the Central Nervous System

Many viruses from different families are called neurotropic for their propensity to infect CNS cells and cause several diseases, including meningitis, encephalitis and meningoencephalitis (see Table 1). Encephalitis is an inflammation of the parenchyma, while meningitis is an inflammation of the leptomeninges. Although these infections may occur together and the spectrum of agents and syndromes overlap, in this chapter we will focus on viral encephalitis.

Viral encephalitis is most commonly caused by herpesviruses, enteroviruses, arboviruses, paramyxoviruses, rhabdoviruses and retroviruses (Griffin, 2003; Johnson, 2003). CNS viral infections may manifest acute, latent or chronic pathology. Viral strain and titer, route of infection, host's age and genetic background (van den Pol, 2009), as well as the extent of CNS injury due to virus-induced neuronal or glial cell death or secondary damage inflicted by immune mediators on infected cells are major factors affecting neuroinvasiveness, tropism, viral clearance or persistency. Most CNS infections present mild symptoms and subjects make a full recovery. Sometimes, however, viral encephalitis may be severe and associated with cell destruction, resulting in permanent brain damage or even death (Chakraborty et al., 2010).

Although herpesviruses (HHV) generally cause asymptomatic infections in humans, they can cause fatal CNS infections in immunocompromised subjects (Griffin, 2003). This is because, following primary exposure, HHV remains latent in the host cell nucleus and can be reactivated if host immune responses fail (Gilden et al., 2007). Herpes simplex virus type 1 and 2 are the etiological agents of acute and sometimes fatal encephalitis (Kleinschmidt-DeMasters and Gilden, 2001). They are capable of infecting not only neurons, but also microglia and astrocytes (Li et al., 2011a). Varicella-Zoster virus has been associated with myelitis, encephalitis and leukoencephalopathy (Gilden et al., 1998). For the Epstein-Barr virus, meningoencephalitis is a recognized complication of infectious mononucleosis, while the cytomegalovirus induces congenital infections associated with a variety of neurological disorders including encephalitis, a condition also observed in immunocompromised subjects

(Landolfo et al., 2003). Astrocytes are a main target and reservoir of HHV-6 in the CNS, which can cause encephalitis in both healthy and immunosuppressed patients (Donati et al., 2005; Johnson, 2003).

**Table 1. Neurotropic viruses associated with human CNS disease**

| Virus | Genus | Family | Genome | Cns disease |
|---|---|---|---|---|
| HSV-1 | Simplexvirus | Herpesviridae | dsDNA | Encephalitis |
| HSV-2 | | | | Encephalitis |
| VZV | Varicellovirus | | | Encephalitis, myelitis and leukoencephalo-pathy |
| EBV | Lymphocrypto-virus | | | Meningoence-phalitis |
| HCMV | Cytomegalovirus | | | Encephalitis |
| HHV-6 | Roseolovirus | | | Encephalitis |
| JCV | Polyomavirus | Polyoma-viridae | dsDNA | Progressive Multifocal Leukoencephalo-pathy |
| Poliovirus | Enterovirus | Picornaviridae | +ssRNA | Poliomyelitis, encephalitis |
| Coxsackie-virus | | | | Encephalitis, mild meningitis |
| ECHO | | | | Encephalitis, mild meningitis |
| EEE Virus[†] | Alphavirus | Togaviridae | | Mild to fatal encephalitis, hemorrhagic syndrome |
| WEE Virus[†] | | | | May be severe in neonates |
| VEE Virus[†] | | | | Mild to fatal encephalomyeli-tis |
| La Crosse[†] | Orthobunyavirus | Bunyaviridae | +ssRNA | Encephalitis |
| JEV[†] | Flavivirus | Flaviviridae | | Encephalitis |
| WNV[†] | | | | Encephalitis, meningitis and acute flaccid paralysis |
| Saint Louis[†] | | | | Mild to severe encephalitis |
| LCMV | Arenavirus | Arenaviridae | -ssRNA | Meningoencephalitis |
| JUNV | | | | Meningoencephalitis |
| MACV | | | | Meningoencephalitis |
| NiV | Henipavirus | Paramyxo-viridae | -ssRNA | Febrile encephalitis |
| Measles Virus | Morbillivirus | | | Meningoencephalitis |
| Mumps Virus | Rubulavirus | | | Meningoencephalitis, aseptic meningitis |
| Rabies Virus | Lyssavirus | Rhabdoviridae | -ssRNA | Acute encephalitis |
| HIV | Lentivirus | Retroviridae | +ssRNA (RT) | Acute or chronic meningitis and encephalitis |
| HTLV-1 | Deltaretrovirus | | | Tropical Spastic Paraparesis / HTLV associated myelopathy |
| HTLV-2 | | | | Subacute myelopathy |

[†] Arbovirus; HSV: Herpes simplex virus; VZV: Varicella-Zoster virus; EBV: Epstein-Bar virus; HCMV: Human cytomegalovirus; HHV-6: Human herpes virus-6; EEE: Eastern equine encephalitis virus; WEE: Western equine encephalitis virus; VEE: Venezuelan equine encephalitis virus; JEV: Japanese encephalitis virus; WNV: West Nile encephalitis virus; LCMV: Lymphocytic choriomeningitis virus; JUNV: Junin virus; MACV: Machupo virus; NiV: Nipah virus; HIV: Human immunodeficiency virus; HTLV: Human T- lymphotropic virus.

The JC virus or John Cunningham virus (JCV), a human polyomavirus that also remains latent, is selective for astrocytes and oligodendrocytes and following reactivation by immunosuppression, elicits a lytic infection and causes progressive multifocal leukoencephalitis (Seth et al., 2004). Usually, enteroviruses, including polioviruses (PV), coxsackieviruses and echoviruses, cause mild meningitis, but sometimes may induce acute encephalitis. PV particularly targets the alpha motor neuron of the anterior horn of the spinal cord and causes poliomyelitis (Rhoades et al., 2011). Neurotropic arboviruses are an extensive group of viruses from the *Flaviviridae*, *Togaviridae* and *Bunyaviridae* families transmitted by arthropods or insects to humans, and can cause mild to fatal encephalitis

(Hollidge et al., 2010). Among them are the eastern equine encephalitis virus (EEEV), the Saint Louis encephalitis virus (SLEV), the La Crosse encephalitis virus (LACV), the western equine encephalitis virus (WEEV), the Japanese encephalitis virus (JEV) and the West Nile encephalitis virus (WNV)(Hollidge et al., 2010; McGavern and Kang, 2011; Schoneboom et al., 1999). Although they are usually associated with viral hemorrhagic fevers, many members of the *Arenaviridae* family can cause neurological disease in humans, including the lymphocytic choriomeningitis virus (LCMV), the Junin virus (JUNV) and the Machupo virus (MACV) (Gómez et al., 2011).

The Nipah virus (NiV), a highly virulent henipavirus of the *Paramyxoviridae* family, may induce severe neurological manifestations, including encephalitis (Johnson, 2003). Measles and mumps viruses, the other members of the *Paramyxoviridae* family, are known to present symptoms such as meningitis and encephalitis (Palacios et al., 2005). However, these neurological diseases are limited to complications of the normal course of the viral infection, with the exception of the rare and fatal subacute sclerosing panencephalitis (Manning et al., 2011). During the acute and fatal encephalitis produced by the rabies virus, a member of the *Rhabdoviridae* family, astrocytes are spared although the proliferation of uninfected reactive astrocytes is an inevitable result of rabies virus-associated encephalomyelitis (Griffin, 2003; Sofroniew and Vinters, 2010). Members of the *Retroviridae* family, such as the human immunodeficiency virus (HIV), can cause latent infection of CNS cells because of their capacity to integrate into the host genome (Lepoutre et al., 2009). Furthermore, the perpetuation strategies of retroviruses include oligoclonal proliferation within the cell that makes viral infection difficult to eradicate (Mortreux et al., 2001). Although HIV mainly targets $CD4^+$ T-cells, it is also a neurotropic virus that has been isolated from cerebrospinal fluid, spinal cord and brain. HIV entry into the CNS may result in several neurological manifestations including acute or chronic encephalitis (McArthur et al., 2005). HIV-1 can infect a small fraction of astrocytes *in vivo*, while productive infection of astrocytes with HIV-1 has significant effects on cell physiology *in vitro* (Cosenza-Nashat et al., 2006; Kim et al., 2004) and is associated with measurable neuropathology in mouse models (Dou et al., 2006). This suggests that infected astrocytes, although infrequent, can have localized pathogenic effects (Borjabad et al., 2010). Astrocyte dysfunction is regarded as the most likely mechanism mediating HIV-related cognitive impairment and neurodegeneration (Wang et al., 2004). HTLV-1 is a T-lymphotropic retrovirus that has been implicated in a distinct neurological disorder termed tropical spastic paraparesis/HTLV-1 associated myelopathy (TSP/HAM), a chronic and progressive debilitating disease of the CNS with particular damage of the corticospinal tracts. TSP/HAM is characterized by an intense proliferation of chronically activated circulating cytotoxic T lymphocytes (CTL)(Mahieux and Gessain, 2007). HTLV-1-infected T lymphocytes impair catabolism and uptake of glutamate in astrocytes via Tax-1 and tumor necrosis factor α (TNF-α)(Szymocha et al., 2000).

Many animal viruses that result in chronic infections of the CNS have been extensively used as models for examining various pathogenic mechanisms, including the roles of astrocyte. Neurons are the main targets in the murine CNS for many kinds of viruses, including Sindbis virus (SINV), a member of the alphaviruses used as a model system for studying viral encephalitis, JEV, WNV, VSV, LCMV and JUNV (Chakraborty et al., 2010; Gómez et al., 2011; Kang and McGavern, 2008). Viruses that cause chronic infection along with myelin loss include the picornavirus Theiler's murine encephalomyelitis virus (TMEV)(Jakob and Roos, 1996), where astrocytes are the major viral reservoirs (Zheng et al.,

2001), the coronavirus mouse hepatitis virus (MHV)(Bergmann et al., 2006) and the paramyxovirus canine distemper virus (CDV)(Wyss-Fluehmann et al., 2010). Finally, experimental rat infections with the Borna disease virus (BDV) have extensively been used to explore viral-induced psychiatric diseases (Ludwig and Bode, 2000).

## Astrocytes Are Activated during Viral Infection

Astrocytes are the most abundant cells in the CNS and increasing evidence points towards their functional heterogeneity from different regions of the CNS (Yeh et al., 2009). In general, they are involved in the regulation of the CNS microenvironment, metabolic support of neurons, synaptic transmission, neurotropism, detoxification, development and maintenance of the BBB, guidance of neuronal migration during development, and several inflammatory and immune functions (Norenberg, 2005; Sidoryk-Wegrzynowicz et al., 2011; Sofroniew and Vinters, 2010).

In several, if not all, forms of CNS injury, including viral CNS infections, astrocytes undergo a dramatic transformation referred to as reactive astrocytosis or astrogliosis (Norenberg, 2005; Sofroniew, 2009). Astrogliosis vary with the nature and severity of the insult in terms of a graduated continuum of progressive alterations in molecular expression, progressive cellular hypertrophy and, in severe cases, proliferation and scar formation (Sofroniew, 2009). It should be differentiated from gliosis or reactive gliosis, which is also frequent in viral infections and includes other cells besides astrocytes such as microglia, macrophages, oligodendroglial progenitor cells, meningeal cells and mesenchymal elements (Norenberg, 2005). When the injury is focal but includes significant necrosis, astrogliosis usually occurs at the margin rather than at the cavitated center of the lesion. Depending on the distance from the lesion, two electrophysiologically, immunohistochemically and morphologically distinct types of hypertrophied astrocytes may be found (Anderova et al., 2001). If the lesion is relatively small, the cavitation it could be fulfilled by reactive astrocytes. In viral infections of the CNS without a cavitary component, astrogliosis may be disseminated (Norenberg, 2005) of the isomorphic type (Fernaud-Espinosa et al., 1993).

Reactive astrocytes exhibit hypertrophy with cytoplasmic processes that are more numerous, longer and thicker. These correlate with an enhanced expression of many proteins, most notably the components of the 10-nm intermediate filaments of the cytoskeleton glial fibrillary acid protein (GFAP)(Eng et al., 2000), vimentin (Lazarides, 1982) and nestin (Lendahl et al., 1990), the last two being expressed only during development and not in most adult astrocytes. Glial activation during CNS viral infection may be triggered in several ways, such as direct viral infection, released viral particles, viral proteins, dsRNA, viral replication and neuronal cell death, as well as other immune challenges (Chen et al., 2010). It is accepted that microglia plays a critical role in the induction of reactive astrogliosis (Giulian et al., 1994; Zhang et al., 2010). Their release of several proinflammatory molecules, including the cytokines interleukin 1 (IL-1), IL-6, TNF-α and IFN-γ, favor astrogliosis, while IL-10 diminishes their extension (Yong, 1996). Many other molecules such as growth factors, neurotransmitters, products associated with neurodegeneration (e.g., prion proteins) and regulators of cell proliferation (e.g., endothelin-1) have been proposed as triggers of astrogliosis (Norenberg, 2005; Sofroniew and Vinters, 2010). Interesting, studies in transgenic mice have revealed that the activation of the endogenous GFAP gene as a consequence of viral infection could involve different regulatory pathways other than activation as a result of prion infection (Titeux et al., 2002). In this regard, a major role in the induction of GFAP has been assigned to nitric oxide (NO)(Brahmachari et al., 2006). Since the inducible form of NO synthase (iNOS), the isoform that produces the highest levels of NO, may be induced by several molecules mentioned above produced by activated microglia and astrocytes (Hewett et al., 1993), it is plausible that NO derived from iNOS might be a relevant mediator of astrocyte activation in processes such as viral infections (Akaike and Maeda, 2000; Munoz-Fernandez and Fresno, 1998; Saha and Pahan, 2006).

Astrogliosis is clearly detected approximately 7 to 10 days after an acute injury, with a peak at 14 to 21 days and a variable time of regression (Norenberg, 2005). In viral infections, it has been observed over much longer periods and may be related to the elimination of the etiologic trigger (Caccuri et al., 2003; Mrak and Griffin, 1997; Wyss-Fluehmann et al., 2010). Reactive astrocytes seem to revert to a more immature stage (Norenberg, 2005; Pekny, 2001). As mentioned before, reactive astrocytes express nestin, vimentin and tenascin-C as well as the neuronal markers MAP-2 (Lin and Matesic, 1994), GABA (Lin et al., 1993), neuron-specific enolase (Lin and Matesic, 1994) and calbindin-D28K (Freund et al., 1990).

Reactive astrocytes show enhanced expression of ion channels ($K^+$, $Ca^{++}$) (Westenbroek et al., 1998), the glutamate transporters GLT-1 and GLAST (Anderson and Swanson, 2000), and the glucose transporter GLUT1 (Norenberg, 2005). They also display gap junctions in their membranes (Landis and Reese, 1981), a fact that could be important in the spreading of viral infections by cell-to-cell transmission. In addition to the mentioned molecules, reactive astrocytes produce a plethora of factors, including enzymes, growth factors, cytokines, extracellular matrix components, protease inhibitors, proto-oncogenes, heat-shock proteins and galectins among many others (Jeon et al., 2010; Norenberg, 2005). Another interesting aspect of astrogliosis is the potential of stem cell production following brain injury, because some astrocytes labeled before injury acquire the capacity to form multipotent and self-renewing neurospheres and may act as a promising source of multipotent cells within the injury site that may be particularly suited to elicit neuronal repair in brain regions far away from zones of adult neurogenesis (Robel et al., 2011). However, the role and utility of such an event in viral infections is still completely unknown.

## Role of Astrocytes in the Innate Viral Immune Response

The absence of lymphatic irrigation, the low levels of major histocompatibility complex (MHC) molecules and the presence of a BBB all enable the CNS to be an immune-privileged organ system (Galea et al., 2007). Astrocyte foot processes are in close opposition to the abluminal surface of the microvascular endothelium of the BBB; thus, astrocytes contribute to both the structural and functional integrity of the BBB (Dong and Benveniste, 2001). In the uninfected CNS, astrocytes and meningeal cells suppress activation of the surrounding cells by producing the anti-inflammatory cytokine transforming growth factor-β (TGF-β)(Griffin, 2003). Toll-like receptors (TLR) 3, 7, 8 and 9 are engaged in viral pathogen-associated molecular pattern recognition and at least TLR 3, 7 and 9 are expressed in activated microglia and astrocytes (Bsibsi et al., 2002; Farina et al., 2005; McKimmie et al., 2005; Suh et al., 2009). They are crucial for the induction of innate and adaptive immune responses within the CNS to protect neuronal cells from invading viruses (Dong and Benveniste, 2001). For example, in human fetal astrocytes, activation of TLR3 by its ligand poly I:C activates more than 1,000 genes including the interferon (IFN)-stimulated genes (ISG)(Rivieccio et al., 2006). Poly I:C-conditioned medium, but not LPS-conditioned medium, promotes the survival of neurons in organotypic human brain slice cultures, implying that TLR3, but not TLR4, binding may elicit neuroprotective gene expression in astrocytes (Bsibsi et al., 2006). In addition, TMEV infection induces TLR3-dependent up-regulation of TLR2, which is critical for the production of proinflammatory molecules (So and Kim, 2009). The production of chemokines in the brain parenchyma acts as a signal to attract pathogen-specific $CD4^+$ and $CD8^+$ T-cells to the CNS and therefore, contributes to the immune-mediated adaptive response to control infection (Kamperschroer and Quinn, 2002). Some studies have also suggested that inappropriate activation of TLR can result in a pathogenic outcome rather than a protective one. Since TLR ligands are actively considered for their antiviral and potential adjuvant effects, this will be an important issue to address in the context of the CNS environment (Suh et al., 2009).

After viral infection of the CNS, a rapid production of type I interferon (IFN I) is critical to inhibit viral spread (Griffin, 2003). Cultured astrocytes infected by TMEV can trigger IFN-α synthesis (So and Kim, 2009). However, in experimental CNS infection by MHV, the main IFN I produced in the CNS is IFN-β, which is produced by macrophages and microglia, but not by neurons or astrocytes (Roth-Cross et al., 2008). This is particularly relevant because preferential production of IFN-β rather than IFN-α is associated with both anti-inflammatory and neuroprotective responses. The anti-inflammatory response, either by direct action or through the induction of anti-inflammatory cytokines such as IL-10, is exerted by down-regulating the expression of molecules such as MHC class II and co-stimulatory molecules, or adhesion molecules, chemokines and matrix metalloproteinases that modulate antigen presentation and trafficking of inflammatory cells into the CNS, respectively (Yong, 2002). The neuroprotective action of IFN-β is less clear and has been associated with either the direct action or through the induction of neurotropic factors (Kieseier and Hartung, 2007). In both the anti-inflammatory and neuroprotective responses, astrocytes have been assigned a critical role (Kieseier and Hartung, 2007; Yong, 2002).

## Role of Astrocytes in the Adaptive Viral Immune Response

Under viral infections, different leukocytes including lymphocytes are capable of invading the CNS. Astrocytes, given their strategic position in the BBB, play a crucial role in limiting the entry of different immune cell subsets into the CNS (Ambrosini et al., 2005). The expression of MHC class II molecules is necessary to induce immune responses through presenting processed antigens to $CD4^+$ T-helper cells. Although MHC class II molecules are usually expressed by specialized antigen-presenting cells (APC) such as B cells, macrophages and dendritic cells, expression on other cell types can be induced by cytokines such as IFN-γ (Dong and Benveniste, 2001). Reactive astrocytes can express class I (Suzumura et al., 1986) and class II (Frank et al., 1986) MHC molecules. Intrathecal injection of IFN-γ induces class II MHC expression in astrocytes, although expression is less intense and occurs later than in microglia (Vass and Lassmann, 1990). Reactive astrocytes also express co-stimulatory molecules B7 and CD40 that are critical for antigen presentation and T-cell activation (Tan et al., 1998) and several studies have showed that reactive astrocytes can effectively process and present antigens to $CD4^+$ T-helper cells (Seth and Koul, 2008), thus maintaining activated Th1 and Th17 cells (Constantinescu et al., 2005). These results led to the proposal that astrocytes function as APC. However, by contrast, other studies in human astrocytes have not found any evidence of expression of CD80 (B7-1), CD86 (B7-2) or CD40 co-stimulating signal molecules (Dong and Benveniste, 2001; Satoh et al., 1995; Windhagen et al., 1995), making the role of astrocytes as APC unclear. Currently, although still controversial, it is proposed that astrocytes may act as APC, but lesser efficiently than microglia (Chastain et al., 2011). The expression of the chemokine CXCL10, associated with the severity of LCMV-induced disease, initially depends on signaling through the IFN I receptor by resident cells, while late expression and up-regulation requires IFN II produced by the recruited $CD8^+$ T-cells. Throughout LCMV infection, the producers of CXCL10 are exclusively resident cells of the CNS, and astrocytes, not microglial cells, are the dominant producers in the neural parenchyma. Based on these results, a model of bidirectional interplay between resident cells of the CNS and the recruited virus-specific T cells with astrocytes as active participants in the local antiviral host response have been suggested (Christensen et al., 2009). Perhaps more studies based on this bidirectional interplay may help to elucidate the *in vivo* role of astrocytes as APC in CNS viral infection.

## Significance of Astrocyte Activation in Viral Infections

The significance of astrogliosis is still unclear (Norenberg, 2005). On one hand, it is generally accepted that reactive astrocytes are beneficial since they exert vital functions that are altered during injury, including restoration of the extracellular microenvironment by removing toxic molecules such as glutamate and free radicals and restoring the BBB (Ridet et al., 1997). They may also participate in axonal and neurite growth by synthesizing several growth factors and extracellular matrix components to facilitate repair and regeneration (Buffo et al., 2008; Norenberg, 2005; Ridet et al., 1997; Sofroniew and Vinters, 2010). This concept is supported by many non-viral and viral studies. In pioneering studies carried out in adult mice expressing HSV-TK under the GFAP promoter and treated with ganciclovir to selectively suppress reactive astrocytes adjacent to a forebrain stab injury, a prolonged infiltration of leukocytes, failure of BBB repair, extensive glutamate-mediated neuronal degeneration and a pronounced increase in local neurite outgrowth was observed, showing a more beneficial than detrimental role of astrogliosis (Bush et al., 1999). Moreover, inhibition of reactive astrocytosis by inducing experimental autoimmune encephalomyelitis (EAE) leads to increased macrophage, but not T cell, infiltration and enhanced severity of EAE (Toft-Hansen et al., 2011). Relatively similar results were found in mice genetically deficient in GFAP and vimentin after a traumatic injury where intermediate filaments of reactive astrocytes were required for proper organization of post-traumatic glial scars (Pekny, 2001).

In JUNV-induced encephalitis and despite heavy infection of neural structures, neurons do not usually show major changes. By contrast, a severe astrocyte reaction is present, showing enhanced expression of GFAP (Lascano and Berria, 1983), iNOS, mitochondrial superoxide dismutase (Gomez et al., 2003) and galectin-3 (Giusti et al., 2011). In chronically infected animals, no correlation between viral antigen and reactive astrocyte distribution has been observed (Lascano et al., 1989). Evidence of a protective role for enhanced NO production is thought not to be related to reduced viral replication but rather to enhanced astrocyte activation, suggesting that this behavior may represent a beneficial cell response to virus-induced CNS damage (Gomez et al., 2003). In HIV-related CNS disease, the protective role of astrocytes seems to be complex. HIV-1 neuroinvasion occurs early (during the period of initial viremia), leading to infection of a limited number of susceptible cells with low CD4 expression. Activation of microglia and astrocytes, due to local or peripheral triggers, increases chemokine production, enhances traffic of infected cells into the CNS and significantly augments the spread of viral species (Persidsky and Poluektova, 2006). The mechanism of HIV-mediated neurologic disorders is not entirely clear, but it is likely to be driven by both direct (active viral replication) and indirect effects of HIV invasion of the brain. Indirect mechanisms include dysregulation of glia, release of viral proteins and elevation of neurotoxic proteins (TNF-α, IL-6, IL-1b, TGF-β, endothelin and glutamate) from resident brain cells and infiltrating lymphocytes (Li et al., 2011b). Glutamate toxicity acts via two distinct pathways: an excitotoxic one, in which glutamate receptors are hyperactivated, and an oxidative one, in which cysteine uptake is inhibited, resulting in glutathione depletion, oxidative stress and cell degeneration. A number of studies have shown that astrocytes normally take up glutamate, keeping extracellular glutamate concentration low in the brain and preventing excitotoxicity. Astrocytes also provide the trophic amino acid glutamine via their expression of glutamine synthetase. These protective and trophic actions are inhibited in HIV infection, probably as a result of the effects of inflammatory mediators and viral proteins (Gras et al., 2006).

On the other hand, astrogliosis can be viewed as detrimental for neuronal function and regeneration by the formation of glial scars (Chvatal et al., 2008; Dong and Benveniste, 2001). In fact, various regeneration inhibitory molecules are synthesized by reactive astrocytes including tenascin-C, chondroitin sulfate proteoglycan, NG2-proteoglycan, matrix metalloproteinases (MMP) and other mechanisms that are not yet fully understood (Chen et al., 2010; Fawcett and Asher, 1999).

It has been demonstrated that WNV infection in astrocytes elicits multiple MMP, which disrupts the BBB, as well as cyclooxygenase enzymes that, by their product prostaglandin E2, regulates the production of multiple inflammatory molecules (Verma et al., 2011). Neuronal apoptosis occurs not only in areas of CNS positive for VEE-antigen, but also in areas of astrogliosis. These findings suggest that the inflammatory response, which is in part mediated by iNOS and TNF-α, may contribute to neurodegeneration following encephalitic viral infection (Schoneboom et al., 2000). In the same line, since TMEV infection of cultured astrocytes induces proinflammatory cytokines, a contribution of activated astrocytes to TMEV-induced demyelinating disease has been proposed (Palma et al., 2003). Moreover, SINV infection leads to changes characteristic of astrogliosis and this reaction has been associated with the pathogenesis of SINV-induced encephalitis by enhancing the local immune response in the CNS (Brodie et al., 1997). Indirect mechanisms have also been implicated. Activated astrocytes are potent producers of IL-6 in the diseased CNS (Dong and

Benveniste, 2001). IL-6 is induced in the brain later than IFN-γ and IL-1 following LCMV infection of mice, consistent with IL-6 exerting its major effect later in the infection course, which contributes to the neurodegenerative signs present in the chronic disease (Kamperschroer and Quinn, 2002).

## Conclusion

Although significant progress has been made in recent years to better understand astrogliosis, the most common and ubiquitous response to CNS injury, the role of astrogliosis in CNS viral infections is still not known. Bearing in mind the contradictory roles of vital or detrimental assigned to it, much more information is still critically needed. Moreover, future studies should include the complex influence of neurons, astrocytes and microglia and vice versa *in vivo* (Rock et al., 2004).

## Acknowledgments

This work was supported by grants from Agencia Nacional de Promoción Científica y Tecnológica (ANPCyT) PICT 07-00642 and PICT 07-00028 (RMG).

## References

Akaike, T., and Maeda, H. (2000). Nitric oxide and virus infection. *Immunology* 101, 300-308.
Ambrosini, E., Remoli, M. E., Giacomini, E., Rosicarelli, B., Serafini, B., Lande, R., Aloisi, F., and Coccia, E. M. (2005). Astrocytes produce dendritic cell-attracting chemokines in vitro and in multiple sclerosis lesions. *J Neuropathol Exp Neurol* 64, 706-715.
Anderova, M., Kubinova, S., Mazel, T., Chvatal, A., Eliasson, C., Pekny, M., and Sykova, E. (2001). Effect of elevated K(+), hypotonic stress, and cortical spreading depression on astrocyte swelling in GFAP-deficient mice. *Glia 35*, 189-203.
Anderson, C. M., and Swanson, R. A. (2000). Astrocyte glutamate transport: review of properties, regulation, and physiological functions. *Glia 32*, 1-14.
Bergmann, C. C., Lane, T. E., and Stohlman, S. A. (2006). Coronavirus infection of the central nervous system: host-virus stand-off. *Nat Rev Microbiol* 4, 121-132.
Borjabad, A., Brooks, A. I., and Volsky, D. J. (2010). Gene expression profiles of HIV-1-infected glia and brain: toward better understanding of the role of astrocytes in HIV-1-associated neurocognitive disorders. *J Neuroimmune Pharmacol 5*, 44-62.
Brahmachari, S., Fung, Y. K., and Pahan, K. (2006). Induction of glial fibrillary acidic protein expression in astrocytes by nitric oxide. *J Neurosci 26*, 4930-4939.
Brodie, C., Weizman, N., Katzoff, A., Lustig, S., and Kobiler, D. (1997). Astrocyte activation by Sindbis virus: expression of GFAP, cytokines, and adhesion molecules. *Glia* 19, 275-285.

Bsibsi, M., Persoon-Deen, C., Verwer, R. W., Meeuwsen, S., Ravid, R., and Van Noort, J.M. (2006). Toll-like receptor 3 on adult human astrocytes triggers production of neuroprotective mediators. *Glia* 53, 688-695.

Bsibsi, M., Ravid, R., Gveric, D., and van Noort, J. M. (2002). Broad expression of Toll-like receptors in the human central nervous system. *J Neuropathol Exp Neurol* 61, 1013-1021.

Buffo, A., Rite, I., Tripathi, P., Lepier, A., Colak, D., Horn, A. P., Mori, T., and Gotz, M. (2008). Origin and progeny of reactive gliosis: A source of multipotent cells in the injured brain. *Proc Natl Acad Sci USA* 105, 3581-3586.

Bush, T. G., Puvanachandra, N., Horner, C. H., Polito, A., Ostenfeld, T., Svendsen, C. N., Mucke, L., Johnson, M. H., and Sofroniew, M. V. (1999). Leukocyte infiltration, neuronal degeneration, and neurite outgrowth after ablation of scar-forming, reactive astrocytes in adult transgenic mice. *Neuron* 23, 297-308.

Caccuri, R. L., Iacono, R. F., Weissenbacher, M. C., Avila, M. M., and Berria, M. I. (2003). Long-lasting astrocyte reaction to persistent Junin virus infection of rat cortical neurons. *J Neural Transm* 110, 847-857.

Chakraborty, S., Nazmi, A., Dutta, K., and Basu, A. (2010). Neurons under viral attack: victims or warriors? *Neurochem Int* 56, 727-735.

Chastain, E. M., Duncan, D. S., Rodgers, J. M., and Miller, S. D. (2011). The role of antigen presenting cells in multiple sclerosis. *Biochim Biophys Acta* 1812, 265-274.

Chen, C. J., Ou, Y. C., Lin, S. Y., Raung, S. L., Liao, S. L., Lai, C. Y., Chen, S. Y., and Chen, J. H. (2010). Glial activation involvement in neuronal death by Japanese encephalitis virus infection. *J Gen Virol* 91, 1028-1037.

Christensen, J. E., Simonsen, S., Fenger, C., Sorensen, M. R., Moos, T., Christensen, J. P., Finsen, B., and Thomsen, A. R. (2009). Fulminant lymphocytic choriomeningitis virus-induced inflammation of the CNS involves a cytokine-chemokine-cytokine-chemokine cascade. *J Immunol* 182, 1079-1087.

Chvatal, A., Anderova, M., Neprasova, H., Prajerova, I., Benesova, J., Butenko, O., and Verkhratsky, A. (2008). Pathological potential of astroglia. *Physiol Res* 57 Suppl 3, S101-110.

Constantinescu, C. S., Tani, M., Ransohoff, R. M., Wysocka, M., Hilliard, B., Fujioka, T., Murphy, S., Tighe, P. J., Das Sarma, J., Trinchieri, G. et al. (2005). Astrocytes as antigen-presenting cells: expression of IL-12/IL-23. *J Neurochem* 95, 331-340.

Cosenza-Nashat, M. A., Si, Q., Zhao, M. L., and Lee, S.C. (2006). Modulation of astrocyte proliferation by HIV-1: differential effects in productively infected, uninfected, and Nef-expressing cells. *J Neuroimmunol* 178, 87-99.

Donati, D., Martinelli, E., Cassiani-Ingoni, R., Ahlqvist, J., Hou, J., Major, E.O., and Jacobson, S. (2005). Variant-specific tropism of human herpesvirus 6 in human astrocytes. *J Virol* 79, 9439-9448.

Dong, Y., and Benveniste, E.N. (2001). Immune function of astrocytes. *Glia* 36, 180-190.

Dou, H., Morehead, J., Bradley, J., Gorantla, S., Ellison, B., Kingsley, J., Smith, L. M., Chao, W., Bentsman, G., Volsky, D. J. et al. (2006). Neuropathologic and neuroinflammatory activities of HIV-1-infected human astrocytes in murine brain. *Glia* 54, 81-93.

Eng, L. F., Ghirnikar, R. S., and Lee, Y. L. (2000). Glial fibrilary acidic protein: GFAP-thirty-one years (1969-2000). *Neurochemical Research* 25, 1439-1451.

Farina, C., Krumbholz, M., Giese, T., Hartmann, G., Aloisi, F., and Meinl, E. (2005). Preferential expression and function of Toll-like receptor 3 in human astrocytes. *J Neuroimmunol* 159, 12-19.

Fawcett, J. W., and Asher, R. A. (1999). The glial scar and central nervous system repair. *Brain Res Bull* 49, 377-391.

Fernaud-Espinosa, I., Nieto-Sampedro, M., and Bovolenta, P. (1993). Differential activation of microglia and astrocytes in aniso- and isomorphic gliotic tissue. *Glia 8*, 277-291.

Frank, E., Pulver, M., and de Tribolet, N. (1986). Expression of class II major histocompatibility antigens on reactive astrocytes and endothelial cells within the gliosis surrounding metastases and abscesses. *J Neuroimmunol* 12, 29-36.

Freund, T. F., Buzsaki, G., Leon, A., Baimbridge, K.G., and Somogyi, P. (1990). Relationship of neuronal vulnerability and calcium binding protein immunoreactivity in ischemia. *Exp Brain Res* 83, 55-66.

Galea, I., Bechmann, I., and Perry, V. H. (2007). What is immune privilege (not)? *Trends Immunol* 28, 12-18.

Gilden, D. H., Bennett, J. L., Kleinschmidt-De Masters, B. K., Song, D. D., Yee, A. S., and Steiner, I. (1998). The value of cerebrospinal fluid antiviral antibody in the diagnosis of neurologic disease produced by varicella zoster virus. *J Neurol Sci* 159, 140-144.

Gilden, D. H., Mahalingam, R., Cohrs, R. J., and Tyler, K. L. (2007). Herpesvirus infections of the nervous system. *Nat Clin Pract Neurol* 3, 82-94.

Giulian, D., Li, J., Li, X., George, J., and Rutecki, P. A. (1994). The impact of microglia-derived cytokines upon gliosis in the CNS. *Dev Neurosci* 16, 128-136.

Giusti, C. J., Alberdi, L., Frik, J., Ferrer, M. F., Scharrig, E., Schattner, M., and Gómez, R.M. (2011). Galectin-3 is upregulated in activated glia during Junín virus-induced murine encephalitis. *Neurosci Lett* 501, 163-166.

Gómez, R. M., Jaquenod de Giusti, C., Sanchez Vallduvi, M. M., Frik, J., Ferrer, M. F., and Schattner, M. (2011). Junín virus. A XXI century update. *Microbes Infect* 13, 303-311.

Gómez, R. M., Yep, A., Schattner, M., and Berria, M. I. (2003). Junín virus-induced astrocytosis is impaired by iNOS inhibition. *J Med Virol* 69, 145-149.

Gras, G., Porcheray, F., Samah, B., and Leone, C. (2006). The glutamate-glutamine cycle as an inducible, protective face of macrophage activation. *J Leukoc Biol* 80, 1067-1075.

Griffin, D. E. (2003). Immune responses to RNA-virus infections of the CNS. *Nat Rev Immunol* 3, 493-502.

Hewett, S. J., Corbett, J. A., McDaniel, M. L., and Choi, D. W. (1993). Interferon-gamma and interleukin-1 beta induce nitric oxide formation from primary mouse astrocytes. *Neurosci Lett* 164, 229-232.

Hollidge, B. S., Gonzalez-Scarano, F., and Soldan, S. S. (2010). Arboviral encephalitides: transmission, emergence, and pathogenesis. *J Neuroimmune Pharmacol 5*, 428-442.

Jakob, J., and Roos, R. P. (1996). Molecular determinants of Theiler's murine encephalomyelitis-induced disease. *J Neurovirol* 2, 70-77.

Jeon, S. B., Yoon, H. J., Chang, C. Y., Koh, H. S., Jeon, S. H., and Park, E. J. (2010). Galectin-3 exerts cytokine-like regulatory actions through the JAK-STAT pathway. *J Immunol* 185, 7037-7046.

Johnson, R. T. (2003). Emerging viral infections of the nervous system. *J Neurovirol* 9, 140-147.

Kamperschroer, C., and Quinn, D. G. (2002). The role of proinflammatory cytokines in wasting disease during lymphocytic choriomeningitis virus infection. *J Immunol* 169, 340-349.

Kang, S. S., and McGavern, D. B. (2008). Lymphocytic choriomeningitis infection of the central nervous system. *Front Biosci* 13, 4529-4543.

Kieseier, B. C., and Hartung, H. P. (2007). Interferon-beta and neuroprotection in multiple sclerosis--facts, hopes and phantasies. *Exp Neurol* 203, 1-4.

Kim, S. Y., Li, J., Bentsman, G., Brooks, A. I., and Volsky, D. J. (2004). Microarray analysis of changes in cellular gene expression induced by productive infection of primary human astrocytes: implications for HAD. *J Neuroimmunol* 157, 17-26.

Kleinschmidt-DeMasters, B. K., and Gilden, D. H. (2001). The expanding spectrum of herpesvirus infections of the nervous system. *Brain Pathol* 11, 440-451.

Landis, D. M., and Reese, T. S. (1981). Membrane structure in mammalian astrocytes: a review of freeze-fracture studies on adult, developing, reactive and cultured astrocytes. *J Exp Biol* 95, 35-48.

Landolfo, S., Gariglio, M., Gribaudo, G., and Lembo, D. (2003). The human cytomegalovirus. *Pharmacol Ther* 98, 269-297.

Lascano, E. F., and Berria, M. I. (1983). Immunoperoxidase study of astrocytic reaction in Junín virus encephalomyelitis of mice. *Acta Neuropathol* 59, 183-190.

Lascano, E. F., Berria, M. I., Avila, M. M., and Weissenbacher, M. C. (1989). Astrocytic reaction predominance in chronic encephalitis of Junín virus-infected rats. *J Med Virol* 29, 327-333.

Lazarides, E. (1982). Intermediate filaments: a chemically heterogeneous, developmentally regulated class of proteins. *Annu Rev Biochem* 51, 219-250.

Lendahl, U., Zimmerman, L. B., and McKay, R. D. (1990). CNS stem cells express a new class of intermediate filament protein. *Cell* 60, 585-595.

Lepoutre, V., Jain, P., Quann, K., Wigdahl, B., and Khan, Z. K. (2009). Role of resident CNS cell populations in HTLV-1-associated neuroinflammatory disease. *Front Biosci* 14, 1152-1168.

Li, J., Hu, S., Zhou, L., Ye, L., Wang, X., Ho, J., and Ho, W. (2011a). Interferon lambda inhibits herpes simplex virus type I infection of human astrocytes and neurons. *Glia* 59, 58-67.

Li, W., Henderson, L. J., Major, E. O., and Al-Harthi, L. (2011b). IFN-gamma mediates enhancement of HIV replication in astrocytes by inducing an antagonist of the beta-catenin pathway (DKK1) in a STAT 3-dependent manner. *J Immunol* 186, 6771-6778.

Lin, R. C., and Matesic, D. F. (1994). Immunohistochemical demonstration of neuron-specific enolase and microtubule-associated protein 2 in reactive astrocytes after injury in the adult forebrain. *Neuroscience* 60, 11-16.

Lin, R. C., Polsky, K., and Matesic, D. F. (1993). Expression of gamma-aminobutyric acid immunoreactivity in reactive astrocytes after ischemia-induced injury in the adult forebrain. *Brain Res* 600, 1-8.

Ludwig, H., and Bode, L. (2000). Borna disease virus: new aspects on infection, disease, diagnosis and epidemiology. *Rev Sci Tech* 19, 259-288.

Mahieux, R., and Gessain, A. (2007). Adult T-cell leukemia/lymphoma and HTLV-1. Curr Hematol *Malig Rep* 2, 257-264.

Manning, L., Laman, M., Edoni, H., Mueller, I., Karunajeewa, H. A., Smith, D., Hwaiwhanje, I., Siba, P. M., and Davis, T. M. (2011). Subacute sclerosing panencephalitis in papua new guinean children: the cost of continuing inadequate measles vaccine coverage. *PLoS Negl Trop Dis* 5, e932.

McArthur, J. C., Brew, B. J., and Nath, A. (2005). Neurological complications of HIV infection. *Lancet Neurol* 4, 543-555.

McGavern, D. B., and Kang, S. S. (2011). Illuminating viral infections in the nervous system. *Nat Rev Immunol* 11, 318-329.

McKimmie, C. S., Johnson, N., Fooks, A. R., and Fazakerley, J. K. (2005). Viruses selectively upregulate Toll-like receptors in the central nervous system. *Biochem Biophys Res Commun* 336, 925-933.

Mortreux, F., Leclercq, I., Gabet, A.S., Leroy, A., Westhof, E., Gessain, A., Wain-Hobson, S., and Wattel, E. (2001). Somatic mutation in human T-cell leukemia virus type 1 provirus and flanking cellular sequences during clonal expansion in vivo. *J Natl Cancer Inst* 93, 367-377.

Mrak, R. E., and Griffin, W. S. (1997). The role of chronic self-propagating glial responses in neurodegeneration: implications for long-lived survivors of human immunodeficiency virus. *J Neurovirol* 3, 241-246.

Munoz-Fernandez, M. A., and Fresno, M. (1998). The role of tumour necrosis factor, interleukin 6, interferon-gamma and inducible nitric oxide synthase in the development and pathology of the nervous system. *Prog Neurobiol* 56, 307-340.

Norenberg, M. D. (2005). The reactive astrocyte. In The Role of Glia in Neurotoxicity, M. Aschner, and L. G. Costa, eds. (CRC), pp. 73-92.

Palacios, G., Jabado, O., Cisterna, D., de Ory, F., Renwick, N., Echevarria, J. E., Castellanos, A., Mosquera, M., Freire, M. C., Campos, R.H., et al. (2005). Molecular identification of mumps virus genotypes from clinical samples: standardized method of analysis. *J Clin Microbiol* 43, 1869-1878.

Palma, J. P., Kwon, D., Clipstone, N. A., and Kim, B. S. (2003). Infection with Theiler's murine encephalomyelitis virus directly induces proinflammatory cytokines in primary astrocytes via NF-kappaB activation: potential role for the initiation of demyelinating disease. *J Virol* 77, 6322-6331.

Pekny, M. (2001). Astrocytic intermediate filaments: lessons from GFAP and vimentin knock-out mice. *Progress in Brain Research* 132, 23-30.

Persidsky, Y., and Poluektova, L. (2006). Immune privilege and HIV-1 persistence in the CNS. *Immunol Rev* 213, 180-194.

Rhoades, R. E., Tabor-Godwin, J. M., Tsueng, G., and Feuer, R. (2011). Enterovirus infections of the central nervous system. *Virology* 411, 288-305.

Ridet, J. L., Malhotra, S. K., Privat, A., and Gage, F. H. (1997). Reactive astrocytes: cellular and molecular cues to biological function. *Trends Neurosci* 20, 570-577.

Rivieccio, M. A., Suh, H. S., Zhao, Y., Zhao, M. L., Chin, K. C., Lee, S. C., and Brosnan, C. F. (2006). TLR3 ligation activates an antiviral response in human fetal astrocytes: a role for viperin/cig5. *J Immunol* 177, 4735-4741.

Robel, S., Berninger, B., and Gotz, M. (2011). The stem cell potential of glia: lessons from reactive gliosis. *Nat Rev Neurosci* 12, 88-104.

Rock, R. B., Gekker, G., Hu, S., Sheng, W. S., Cheeran, M., Lokensgard, J. R., and Peterson, P. K. (2004). Role of microglia in central nervous system infections. *Clin Microbiol Rev* 17, 942-964, table of contents.

Roth-Cross, J. K., Bender, S. J., and Weiss, S. R. (2008). Murine coronavirus mouse hepatitis virus is recognized by MDA5 and induces type I interferon in brain macrophages/microglia. *J Virol* 82, 9829-9838.

Saha, R. N., and Pahan, K. (2006). Regulation of inducible nitric oxide synthase gene in glial cells. *Antioxid Redox Signal* 8, 929-947.

Satoh, J., Lee, Y. B., and Kim, S. U. (1995). T-cell costimulatory molecules B7-1 (CD80) and B7-2 (CD86) are expressed in human microglia but not in astrocytes in culture. *Brain Res* 704, 92-96.

Schoneboom, B. A., Catlin, K. M., Marty, A. M., and Grieder, F. B. (2000). Inflammation is a component of neurodegeneration in response to Venezuelan equine encephalitis virus infection in mice. *J Neuroimmunol* 109, 132-146.

Schoneboom, B. A., Fultz, M. J., Miller, T. H., McKinney, L. C., and Grieder, F. B. (1999). Astrocytes as targets for Venezuelan equine encephalitis virus infection. *J Neurovirol* 5, 342-354.

Seth, P., Diaz, F., Tao-Cheng, J. H., and Major, E. O. (2004). JC virus induces nonapoptotic cell death of human central nervous system progenitor cell-derived astrocytes. *J Virol* 78, 4884-4891.

Seth, P., and Koul, N. (2008). Astrocyte, the star avatar: redefined. *J Biosci* 33, 405-421.

Sidoryk-Wegrzynowicz, M., Wegrzynowicz, M., Lee, E., Bowman, A.B., and Aschner, M. (2011). Role of astrocytes in brain function and disease. *Toxicol Pathol* 39, 115-123.

So, E. Y., and Kim, B. S. (2009). Theiler's virus infection induces TLR3-dependent upregulation of TLR2 critical for proinflammatory cytokine production. *Glia* 57, 1216-1226.

Sofroniew, M. V. (2009). Molecular dissection of reactive astrogliosis and glial scar formation. *Trends Neurosci* 32, 638-647.

Sofroniew, M. V., and Vinters, H. V. (2010). Astrocytes: biology and pathology. *Acta Neuropathol* 119, 7-35.

Suh, H. S., Brosnan, C. F., and Lee, S. C. (2009). Toll-like receptors in CNS viral infections. *Curr Top Microbiol Immunol* 336, 63-81.

Suzumura, A., Lavi, E., Weiss, S. R., and Silberberg, D. H. (1986). Coronavirus infection induces H-2 antigen expression on oligodendrocytes and astrocytes. *Science* 232, 991-993.

Szymocha, R., Akaoka, H., Dutuit, M., Malcus, C., Didier-Bazes, M., Belin, M. F., and Giraudon, P. (2000). Human T-cell lymphotropic virus type 1-infected T lymphocytes impair catabolism and uptake of glutamate by astrocytes via Tax-1 and tumor necrosis factor alpha. *J Virol* 74, 6433-6441.

Tan, L., Gordon, K. B., Mueller, J. P., Matis, L. A., and Miller, S. D. (1998). Presentation of proteolipid protein epitopes and B7-1-dependent activation of encephalitogenic T cells by IFN-gamma-activated SJL/J astrocytes. *J Immunol* 160, 4271-4279.

Titeux, M., Galou, M., Gomes, F. C., Dormont, D., Neto, V.M., and Paulin, D. (2002). Differences in the activation of the GFAP gene promoter by prion and viral infections. *Brain Res Mol Brain Res* 109, 119-127.

Toft-Hansen, H., Fuchtbauer, L., and Owens, T. (2011). Inhibition of reactive astrocytosis in established experimental autoimmune encephalomyelitis favors infiltration by myeloid cells over T cells and enhances severity of disease. *Glia* 59, 166-176.

van den Pol, A. N. (2009). Viral infection leading to brain dysfunction: more prevalent than appreciated? *Neuron* 64, 17-20.

Vass, K., and Lassmann, H. (1990). Intrathecal application of interferon gamma. Progressive appearance of MHC antigens within the rat nervous system. *Am J Pathol* 137, 789-800.

Verma, S., Kumar, M., and Nerurkar, V.R. (2011). Cyclooxygenase-2 inhibitor blocks the production of West Nile virus-induced neuroinflammatory markers in astrocytes. *J Gen Virol* 92, 507-515.

Wang, Z., Trillo-Pazos, G., Kim, S. Y., Canki, M., Morgello, S., Sharer, L. R., Gelbard, H. A., Su, Z. Z., Kang, D. C., Brooks, A. I., et al. (2004). Effects of human immunodeficiency virus type 1 on astrocyte gene expression and function: potential role in neuropathogenesis. *J Neurovirol* 10 *Suppl 1*, 25-32.

Westenbroek, R. E., Bausch, S. B., Lin, R. C., Franck, J. E., Noebels, J. L., and Catterall, W. A. (1998). Upregulation of L-type $Ca^{2+}$ channels in reactive astrocytes after brain injury, hypomyelination, and ischemia. *J Neurosci* 18, 2321-2334.

Windhagen, A., Newcombe, J., Dangond, F., Strand, C., Woodroofe, M. N., Cuzner, M. L., and Hafler, D. A. (1995). Expression of costimulatory molecules B7-1 (CD80), B7-2 (CD86), and interleukin 12 cytokine in multiple sclerosis lesions. *J Exp Med* 182, 1985-1996.

Wyss-Fluehmann, G., Zurbriggen, A., Vandevelde, M., and Plattet, P. (2010). Canine distemper virus persistence in demyelinating encephalitis by swift intracellular cell-to-cell spread in astrocytes is controlled by the viral attachment protein. *Acta Neuropathol* 119, 617-630.

Yeh, T. H., Lee da, Y., Gianino, S. M., and Gutmann, D. H. (2009). Microarray analyses reveal regional astrocyte heterogeneity with implications for neurofibromatosis type 1 (NF1)-regulated glial proliferation. *Glia* 57, 1239-1249.

Yong, V. W. (1996). Cytokines, astrogliosis, and neurotrophism following CNS trauma. In *Cytokines and the CNS*, J. Ransohof, and E.N. Benveniste, eds. (Boca Raton, CRC), pp. 309-327.

Yong, V. W. (2002). Differential mechanisms of action of interferon-beta and glatiramer aetate in MS. *Neurology* 59, 802-808.

Zhang, D., Hu, X., Qian, L., O'Callaghan, J. P., and Hong, J. S. (2010). Astrogliosis in CNS pathologies: is there a role for microglia? *Mol Neurobiol* 41, 232-241.

Zheng, L., Calenoff, M. A., and Dal Canto, M. C. (2001). Astrocytes, not microglia, are the main cells responsible for viral persistence in Theiler's murine encephalomyelitis virus infection leading to demyelination. *J Neuroimmunol* 118, 256-267.

In: Astrocytes
Editor: Oscar González-Pérez

ISBN: 978-1-62081-558-8
© 2012 Nova Science Publishers, Inc.

*Chapter VIII*

# Astrocyte Dysfunction in Megalencephalic Leukoencephalopathy with Subcortical Cysts

*Raúl Estévez*[*]

Physiology section, Department Physiological Sciences II, School of Medicine,
University of Barcelona, Barcelona, Spain
Centro de Investigación en Red de Enfermedades Raras
(CIBERER), ISCIII, Spain

## Abstract

In the normal CNS, astrocytes actively regulate normal brain function. The regulation of processes related to brain homeostasis and myelination seems to be its major task. The role of astrocytes in myelin biology is impressively illustrated by mutations in astrocyte-expressed genes in human leukodystrophies (genetic diseases of the white matter).

We review here Megalencephalic leukoencephalopathy with subcortical cysts (MLC), which is a vacuolating myelinopathy.

The genes affected in this disease code for a membrane protein with low homology to ion channels (MLC1) and an adhesion membrane protein of poorly characterized function (GlialCAM), which acts as an escort molecule of MLC1. In addition, GlialCAM functions as an auxiliary subunit of the chloride channel ClC-2, and ClC-2 knockout mice display an MLC-like phenotype.

We provide here an introduction about this disorder and review the last findings. The study of MLC disease provides new exciting insights about the role of astrocytes in the process of myelin homeostasis.

---

[*] Address: Faculty of Medicine, Department of Physiological Sciences II, Campus de Bellvitge, Pavelló de Govern, C/Feixa Llarga s/n. 08907, L'Hospitalet de Llobregat, Barcelona, Spain. Tel: +34 934039781; Fax: +34 934024268; E-mail: restevez@ub.edu.

## Introduction

Astrocytes are the major glial cells in the central nervous system, defined by their stellate morphology and the expression of several astrocyte-specific genes, including glial fibrillary acid protein (GFAP) (Messing and Brenner, 2003). They play multiple roles organizing and maintaining brain structure and function, and they are essential to support neuronal activity (Attwell et al., 2010; Eroglu and Barres, 2010). One of their principal function is to keep the ionic composition of the extracellular medium constant (Kofuji and Newman, 2004). Thus, ion and water fluxes by channel proteins in astrocytes are important for fluid homeostasis and in maintaining a low extracellular potassium concentration after neuronal repolarization (Neusch et al., 2001). Water and potassium homeostasis seems to be directly linked to each other, as disruption of water channels affects potassium clearance (Amiry-Moghaddam et al., 2003; Amiry-Moghaddam et al., 2004), and concomitantly, disruption of potassium channels also affects water clearance (Haj-Yasein et al., 2011).

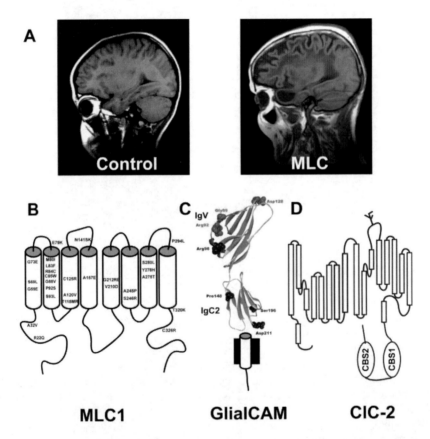

Figure 1. MLC disease and proteins that have been related with the molecular basis of its pathology. (A) A typical MRI image of an MLC patient comparing to a control subject. (B) Predicted 2D model of MLC1 indicating the position of the missense mutations identified until date. (C) Predicted model of GlialCAM indicating the position of the identified recessive missense (blue) and dominant (pink) mutations. (D) 2D model of the ClC-2 chloride channel.

The process of myelination in the central nervous system appeared in the evolution of chordates (Nave, 2010). By this process, axons become insulated, which is conditional to speed up electrical transmission and to reduce energy consumption. Furthermore, it allowed increasing the complexity of the brain while keeping a reduced size. Astrocyte function is also important for normal myelination and to promote re-myelination after an injury in the nervous system. Astrocytes regulate by different mechanisms the myelinating cells, role fulfilled by the oligodendrocytes in the central nervous system (Nave, 2010).

Leukodystrophies comprise a heterogeneous group of degenerative genetic diseases affecting the cerebral white matter (WM, myelin-rich regions of the brain) (Kaye, 2001; Schiffmann and Boespflug-Tanguy, 2001; Schiffmann and van der Knaap, 2004). As expected, pathogenic mutations in several oligodendrocyte-expressed genes have been found in some of these diseases (Kaye, 2001). Interestingly, in several types of leukodystrophies, such as Alexander disease (Messing et al., 2010; Prust et al., 2011) and Megalencephalic leukoencephalopathy with subcortical cysts (MLC) (Leegwater et al., 2001), mutations in two genes expressed mostly in astrocytes and not in oligodendrocytes have also been found (Schmitt et al., 2003). These results highlight the role of astrocytes in myelination. In this chapter, we will review the literature about MLC and discuss new results recently obtained. These new discoveries illustrate the different roles that astrocytes seem to play in brain and myelin homeostasis.

# MLC Disease:
# Clinical and Genetic Characteristics

MLC (MIM, 604004) is a rare form of leukodystrophy (van der Knaap et al., 1995). It shows a relatively mild phenotype characterized by early-onset macrocephalia and delayed-onset ataxia, spasticity, epilepsia and mild mental deterioration. The diagnosis of MLC is established in individuals with typical clinical findings and characteristic abnormalities on brain MRI (Figure 1). A brain biopsy revealed the presence of vacuoles mostly within the outer part of myelin sheaths (van der Knaap et al., 1996). Diffusion studies indicated that there is an increased content of water in the brain, which may explain the megalencephaly (Singhal et al., 2003). There is no therapy available and the treatment is just supportive to ameliorate the symptoms.

The fact that the disease could be precisely diagnosed by the presence of specific MRI patterns and clinical parameters allowed medical doctors to perform genetic linkage studies (Topcu et al., 1998; Topcu et al., 2000). Most patients show a recessive genetic inheritance pattern, it is, two defective copies of the gene are necessary to develop the disease. From linkage studies, the first gene associated with MLC was mapped to chromosome 22qtel (Topcu et al., 2000) and identified as *MLC1* (also called *KIAA0027* or *WKL1*) (Leegwater et al., 2001). Mutations in *MLC1* were approximately found in 70% of the MLC patients (Ilja Boor et al., 2006; Leegwater et al., 2002b; Wang et al., 2011; Yuzbasioglu et al., 2011). However, several patients with the MLC phenotype did not carry mutations in *MLC1*, suggesting the involvement of other genes in the disease (Leegwater et al., 2002b). Further genetic studies indicated that patients without mutations in *MLC1* did not show linkage to the *MLC1* locus, confirming that other unidentified MLC genes may exist (Blattner et al., 2003;

Patrono et al., 2003). In these patients, according with the evolution of the disease at older ages (van der Knaap et al., 2010), two phenotypes can be distinguished: classical MLC and benign MLC. In classical MLC, patients have the same phenotype as the ones carrying *MLC1* mutations, whereas patients with benign MLC show an age-improving phenotype. Moreover, the improving phenotype can be further classified into benign macrocephaly or the clinical syndrome of macrocephaly and mental retardation with or without autism (Lopez-Hernandez et al., 2011a). The presence of these two phenotypes was suggestive of genetic heterogeneity. Furthermore, even in patients with the same *MLC1* mutation, there is intrafamilial variability of the phenotype, indicating that unknown environmental or genetic factors influence the severity of the disease (Pascual-Castroviejo et al., 2005). It was also reported that some amino acid exchanges in MLC1 were associated with catatonic schizophrenia (Meyer et al., 2001; Selch et al., 2007; Verma et al., 2005), although other groups did not support this hypothesis (Devaney et al., 2002; Kaganovich et al., 2004; Leegwater et al., 2002a; Rubie et al., 2003). In agreement with the latter suggestion, an amino acid change (L309M) related with catatonic schizophrenia does not affect MLC1 surface levels (see below) (Teijido et al., 2004). Future work is needed to clarify this issue.

## MLC1 Protein Features

*MLC1* encodes a membrane protein with eight predicted transmembrane domains and intracellular N- and C- termini (Figure 1). Immunofluorescence in MLC1-transfected cells with non-permeabilized conditions using different antibodies proved the intracellular location of both termini (Boor et al., 2005). *MLC1* gene is not present in all phylae, and it is only present in myelin-presenting animals, from teleosts to mammals. There are no other close homologues in the human genome (Leegwater et al., 2001). Sequence comparisons showed that MLC1 has low identity with the Kv1 potassium channels, especially in the voltage sensor area (Teijido et al., 2004). Similar to what happens in other membrane transport proteins, there are regions of internal homology in MLC1 (Teijido et al., 2004). Thus, the transmembrane domains of the first half of the protein showed sequence identity to the second half. The weak identity between the two halves is more evident in the predicted transmembrane domains 4 and 8, which are characterized by a stretch of leucine residues. Poly-leucine segments normally act as an oligomerization interfaces, as have been found in other membrane proteins (Gurezka et al., 1999).

There are several biochemical evidences that suggest that MLC1 form homo-oligomers. First of all, detection of the protein by Western blot recognizes several bands corresponding to its monomeric and dimeric forms (Teijido et al., 2004). It is important to note that MLC1 is detected with a minor molecular weight from what is predicted from its amino acid sequence. This type of behaviour is usually seen in many hydrophobic membrane proteins (Pineda et al., 1999). Secondly, several biochemical studies, including assembly-dependent trafficking assays (Teijido et al., 2004), co-immunoprecipitation and protein complementation assays (Lopez-Hernandez et al., 2011b), have shown that MLC1 is able to homo-oligomerize. Whether MLC1 forms dimers or higher-order structures have to be defined.

MLC1 sequence analysis suggests that there is a putative glycosylation site between transmembrane domains 3 and 4. However, treatment with glycosidases and mutagenesis studies indicated that the protein is not glycosylated (Teijido et al., 2004). Nevertheless, introduction of a loop sequence containing a glycosylation site from an unrelated protein between these two transmembrane domains leads to the glycosylation of MLC1 (Duarri et al., 2008). From a topological point of view, this result indicates that this region is extracellular. Similar results can be extrapolated from the extracellular loop between transmembrane segments 7 and 8, where an HA epitope tag could be inserted and detected from outside of the cell (Teijido et al., 2004).

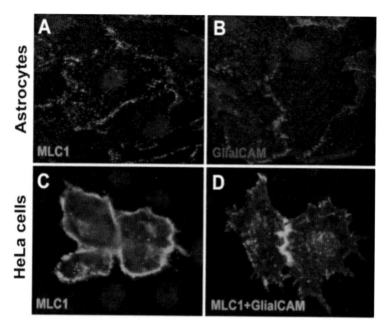

Figure 2. Localization of MLC1 and GlialCAM in astrocyte-astrocyte junctions. GlialCAM as an escort molecule for MLC1 in heterologous cells. Characterization of MLC1 (A) and GlialCAM (B) expression in rat primary astrocytes. Localization is found in cellular processes linking astrocytes co-localizing with adherent and tight junctions proteins. (C) MLC1 expressed in HeLa cells is localized at the plasma membrane, but it is redistributed to HeLa cell junctions after co-expression with GlialCAM (D).

*In vitro* biochemical studies using glutathione-fusion proteins containing the MLC1 N-terminus or the C-terminus expressed in bacteria indicated that both terminal parts are phosphorylated by protein kinase A/C in serine 27, and by protein kinase C in serine 339 (Lanciotti et al., 2010). Treatment with PKA/C activators increases the presence of a 60-kDa band which is suggested to be associated with the plasma membrane, and lead to an increase in the presence of MLC1 in astrocytic processes (Lanciotti et al., 2010). However, it is not clear whether these residues are involved in this effect, since mutagenesis studies mimicking or eliminating the phosphorylation of these two serine residues have not been performed.

Expression of MLC1 alone in heterologous systems (Teijido et al., 2004) revealed its localization at the plasma membrane (Figure 2). MLC1 is also located at the plasma membrane in astrocytes on tissue preparations, but mainly in astrocyte-astrocyte junctions (Teijido et al., 2007).

Thus, as MLC1 is located at the plasma membrane and shows sequence similarity to ion channels, we and others speculated that it could be an ion channel itself (Kaganovich et al., 2004; Leegwater et al., 2001; Teijido et al., 2004). In voltage-clamp studies in *Xenopus* oocytes and patch-clamp experiments in tsA-201 cells, no ion channel activity could be measured (Teijido et al., 2004; Kaganovich et al., 2004). As MLC1 shows identity to Kv1.1, we also co-expressed both proteins, but no changes could be detected in Kv1.1 functional properties (Teijido et al., 2004). Similar studies were also performed using Kir4.1, the main potassium channel of astrocytes, where MLC1 shows higher expression, but no changes in Kir4.1 properties were found after MLC1 co-expression (Teijido et al., 2007). However, very recently, it has been reported that MLC1 expression is related with VRAC (volume-regulated anion channel) activity after expression in HEK and Sf9 cells (Ridder et al., 2011). These results should be taken with caution: they do not indicate that MLC1 is the protein responsible for VRAC activity or even that MLC1 directly regulates this channel, as the expression of many different proteins influences this activity. As a typical example in the VRAC field, expression of pICln (a regulator of small nuclear ribonucleoproteins) also influences VRAC activity (Krapivinsky et al., 1994; Paulmichl et al., 1992; Pu et al., 1999). Thus, although the phenotype observed in MLC patients is still suggestive that MLC1 has a role in ion/water handling across membranes, the function of MLC1 is far from being defined.

## MLC1 Mutations: Molecular Mechanism of Pathogenesis

As our attempts to measure a putative MLC1-mediated electrical activity were unsuccessful, we decided to analyze the biochemical defect caused by missense mutations found in MLC patients. These mutations were introduced in MLC1, and total and plasma membrane levels were analyzed after expression of the defective proteins in heterologous cells (Duarri et al., 2008; Montagna et al., 2006; Teijido et al., 2004). Most disease-causing missense mutations showed a reduction in its total protein levels, and concomitantly a diminished surface expression. By using different biochemical methods, it was demonstrated that this was caused by an increase in the degradation of these defective proteins associated to the proteasomal endoplasmatic reticulum and to the lysosomal degradation machineries (Duarri et al., 2008). A similar surface localization defect was found after expressing some of these defective proteins in primary culture of astrocytes (Duarri et al., 2008).

More importantly, these results could also be validated using human samples obtained from MLC patients. These included monocytes obtained from the blood of patients (Duarri et al., 2008) and from brain tissue of an MLC patient harbouring a missense mutation (Lopez-Hernandez et al., 2011b). Based on these results, we could conclude that *MLC1* mutations reduce protein levels *in vivo*.

Rescue of protein expression was achieved using inhibitors of the proteasome and the lysosomal degradation machinery, improving the folding at low temperatures or using chemical chaperones (Duarri et al., 2008; Teijido et al., 2004). Accordingly, it was suggested that *MLC1* mutations affect the conformation of the protein. As it happens in many other genetic disorders, all strategies to boost MLC1 expression could have a therapeutical use for the disease. However, as the function of MLC1 is not known, restoring protein levels or improving the traffic of the protein to the plasma membrane could not be enough, as the mutated protein may still not be functional.

# MLC1 Localization in Tissue and in Astrocytes

Studies aimed to describe the expression of *MLC1* have been performed in rodent tissue during different stages of development by means of *in situ* hybridization (Schmitt et al., 2003; Teijido et al., 2004) and immunohistochemistry with polyclonal antibodies (Teijido et al., 2004; Teijido et al., 2007), and in human adult tissue by means of immunohistochemistry with polyclonal antibodies (Ambrosini et al., 2008; Boor et al., 2007; Boor et al., 2005; Duarri et al., 2008; Duarri et al., 2011).

All studies performed by different groups have detected *MLC1* mRNA and protein in adult mouse, mostly in Bergmann glial cells in the cerebellum, in ependymal cells surrounding the ventricles, and in astrocytes around perivascular and subpial regions, and several GFAP-positive astrocytes throughout the brain. No expression was found in microglia or oligodendrocytes (Schmitt et al., 2003; Teijido et al., 2004). Similar results were found in human adult tissue (Ambrosini et al., 2008; Boor et al., 2007; Boor et al., 2005; Duarri et al., 2008; Duarri et al., 2011).

In addition, ISH also detected *MLC1* expression in mouse neuronal cell bodies of several brain regions and, furthermore, there was also immunohistochemical staining of particular axonal tracts (Teijido et al., 2004). The pattern of expression in neurons was consistent during development (Teijido et al., 2007). In relative quantities, MLC1 is enriched in mouse astrocytes compared to neurons, so low sensitivity may explain the lack of detection in *MLC1* in mouse neuronal tissue by some laboratories (Schmitt et al., 2003).

However, expression in neurons in human adult tissue was not reported. Thus, it was suggested that MLC could be considered as a leukodystrophy of astrocytic origin (Gorospe and Maletkovic, 2006). Further work is needed to explain the discrepancies between human and mouse expression patterns. With the higher resolutive EM immunogold method in mouse and human tissue (Duarri et al., 2011; Teijido et al., 2007), it was revealed that MLC1 is present in protoplasmatic and perivascular astrocyte-astrocyte junctions, but not in endothelium-astrocyte junctions. Double immunogold EM in human tissue studying MLC1 and β-Dystroglycan, which is located in astrocyte membranes contacting basal lamina, showed that both proteins did not colocalize (Duarri et al., 2011). Thus, we concluded that MLC1 in astrocytes is not a component of the dystrophin-glycoprotein complex (DGC), as is not located in the perivascular membrane, but it is rather in astrocytic processes that link astrocytes to each other. In addition, in the brain from several DGC components null mice no change in MLC1 expression was found (Duarri et al., 2011).

However, other groups using confocal microscopy suggested that MLC1 forms part of the DGC, as it co-localized at the astrocytic endfeet with DGC proteins (Ambrosini et al., 2008; Boor et al., 2007). In view of the small distances between different membranes at and between the endfeet (Mathiisen et al., 2010), this method is not resolutive enough. Other experiments indicating that MLC1 formed part of the DGC were based on biochemical fractionation or co-immunoprecipitation using crosslinking reagents (Ambrosini et al., 2008; Boor et al., 2007). Special care should be taken in these approaches, as MLC1 is a very hydrophobic and sticky protein. In this sense, co-immunoprecipitation studies without crosslinking failed to detect interaction between MLC1 and members of the DGC (Duarri et al., 2011). Interestingly, in work performed with human control brain tissue, brain tissue from an MLC patient and brain tissue from a glioblastoma, it was shown that there was an altered expression of several DGC proteins (Boor et al., 2007). Although we believe that MLC1 perform its physiological function at the plasma membrane in astrocytic junctions, it could be possible that intracellular MLC1 is associated with protein members of the DGC, unifying the discrepancies between the different findings.

Localization studies have also been performed in astrocyte cultures (Ambrosini et al., 2008; Duarri et al., 2011; Lanciotti et al., 2010). In primary rat astrocytes, endogenous MLC1 is detected in a diffuse intracellular staining through the cytoplasm, co-localizing with endoplasmatic reticulum and endosomal markers. Treatment with compounds that block cell proliferation and/or cause cell differentiation led to an increase of protein expression in longer time cultures, but, more importantly, this treatment also led to a re-distribution of MLC1 to astrocyte-astrocyte junctions (Duarri et al., 2011) (Figure 2). This differentiated astrocyte culture was then used as a model for the *in vivo* situation, as it reproduced the protein localization in tissue. In these astrocytic processes, co-localization was observed with components of tight junctions such as *zonula occludens* (ZO-1) or occludin, and components of adherent junctions such as β-catenin or N-cadherin (Duarri et al., 2011). Co-immunoprecipitation and co-localization in tissue by immunogold EM between ZO-1 and MLC1 was also observed. Proteins from the DGC, gap junctions, focal adhesions or developing astrocyte processes do not co-localize with MLC1 in this differentiated cell model (Duarri et al., 2011). In contrast, co-localization with DGC proteins was found in intracellular compartments in the undifferentiated astrocytic model (Ambrosini et al., 2008), supporting the hypothesis that intracellular MLC1 is associated with these proteins. Disruption of the actin cytoskeleton, but not the microtubule or the GFAP network, affected MLC1 localization in junctions. It could be speculated that MLC1 is linked to the actin cytoskeleton via interaction with ZO-1, as ZO-1 works as a scaffold molecule (Fanning and Anderson, 2009).

## Molecular Consequences of the Lack of MLC1

Mutations found in MLC patients reduce MLC1 protein levels. Thus, in order to understand the pathophysiology of MLC disease, different strategies could be used to eliminate or reduce MLC1 protein expression in experimental model systems. The first approach used was lymphoblast cell lines derived from patients. Although northern blot studies showed that *MLC1* was expressed in peripheral blood leukocytes, quantitative real-time PCR of human lymphoblast cell lines showed that these cells expressed about 1000 fold lower amount of *MLC1* mRNA from that is found in the brain (Duarri et al., 2008). In addition, Western blot using specific antibodies directed against human MLC1 failed to detect protein expression in lymphoblast cell lines. Although MLC1 is not detectable, some differences in functional properties have been found between lymphoblast cell lines from patients and controls (Ridder et al., 2011). Alternatively, human monocytes were shown to express MLC1 as well. In addition, MLC1 protein was not present in monocytes from patients, indicating that this model is potentially useful (Duarri et al., 2008). Unfortunately, expression of MLC1 was only detected in fresh blood, limiting the use of this primary cell for further studies (Van der Knaap, personal communication).

As MLC1 is mainly expressed in astrocytes, we selected primary rat cultures of astrocytes and performed RNA interference mediated by adenoviruses (Duarri et al., 2011).

Real-time, western blot and immunofluorescence experiments indicated that *MLC1* mRNA and protein were nearly absent after RNAi expression, strongly validating the specificity of the antibodies used in our work. Cells depleted of MLC1 displayed vacuolation (Duarri et al., 2011). However, vacuoles had been mainly found in myelin in a biopsy from an MLC patient (van der Knaap et al., 1996) and therefore, the significance of this result was not clear. Careful re-examination of the same brain biopsy consistently found vacuoles within perivascular astrocytic endfeet. Then, we can conclude that vacuolation of astrocytes is also a hallmark of MLC disease (Duarri et al., 2011).

Is there any biochemical defect that could explain the observed vacuolation? Electrophysiological studies (Ridder et al., 2011) demonstrated that lymphoblast cell lines from MLC patients and astrocytes with reduced MLC1 expression showed less activity of the volume regulated anion channel (VRAC) (Kimelberg, 2004). VRAC is responsible of chloride and osmolyte efflux upon a hypoosmotic shock (Ernest et al., 2005). Water follows these anions in a process named regulatory volume decrease (RVD) (Pasantes-Morales et al., 2006). Convincingly, both cell types showed a slow RVD response. We predict that as the water is a highly reactive reagent, if cells are unable to drive the excess out of their citoplasm, it will be encapsulated into vacuoles, in a similar manner to what have been described in lower organisms (Becker et al., 1999). Thus, a decrease in VRAC activity in MLC could potentially explain the presence of vacuoles in astrocytes. But, how are vacuoles formed in myelin? It might be that vacuoles appear in myelin due to non-cell autonomous effects, but additional experiments are needed to clarify this issue. Although the decrease in VRAC activity is the first functional defect found in MLC disease (Ridder et al., 2011), the relationship between MLC1 and VRAC activity is unknown, as this channel is regulated at multiple levels.

## MLC1 Protein Network and the Identification of a Second MLC Disease Gene

In order to get insight into the MLC1 role, we and others tried to identify interacting proteins (Brignone et al., 2011; Lopez-Hernandez et al., 2011a). This type of methodology is challenging for membrane proteins. For instance, immunoprecipitation assays need the disruption of the biological samples and the solubilization of the membrane proteins, which may disrupt these interactions or even create additional ones by unspecific aggregation, leading to potential artifacts. In order to avoid these unwanted pitfalls, correlative quantitative proteomic after affinity purification was performed using three different antibodies directed against MLC1 (Lopez-Hernandez et al., 2011a). Protein abundance determined that GlialCAM was the second protein with the highest yield (after MLC1) in all purifications. Interaction between both proteins was direct, as it could be reproduced after transfection in heterologous cells and detection of the interaction by co-immunoprecipitation, FRET or split-TEV experiments (Lopez-Hernandez et al., 2011a; Lopez-Hernandez et al., 2011b).

GlialCAM (also called HepaCAM) (Chung Moh et al., 2005; Moh et al., 2005) is a type I membrane (C terminus intracellular) glycoprotein (Figure 1). In the beginning of the N-terminal part there is a signal peptide, which is cleaved after translation, and two immunoglobulin (Ig) domains, from the types IgV and IgC2. The C-terminus is rich in proline residues and it has been suggested that it is phosphorylated (Moh et al., 2005). *GLIALCAM* was identified as a suppressed gene in hepatic tumours (Chung Moh et al., 2005), although subsequent expression studies in normal tissues found GlialCAM mostly expressed in the brain (Favre-Kontula et al., 2008). As *MLC1*, *GLIALCAM* is only present in myelin-forming organisms, from teleosts to mammals. GlialCAM protein expression increases during development, in a clear parallelism with the formation of myelin (Favre-Kontula et al., 2008). In different cell types, it has been related with functions of cell growth, differentiation, motility and adhesion (He et al., 2010; Lee et al., 2009; Moh et al., 2009a; Moh et al., 2009b; Xun et al., 2010; Zhang et al., 2010). There is a report indicating that a knockout mouse for GlialCAM has been generated, but the phenotype of these mice have not been described (Favre-Kontula et al., 2008). There is a close homologue to GlialCAM, called HepaCAM2, which shows a similar topology, but contains three Ig domains at the N terminus, instead of two. Both proteins are homologous to other cell adhesion molecules belonging to the SLAM family (Engel et al., 2003) with important roles in the immune system. Comparison of the sequence between these proteins in the Ig domains indicates that the residues of the IgC2 domain are more conserved to those from the IgV domain. As the adhesion between different SLAM proteins occur primarily by interaction between the IgV (variable) domains (Engel et al., 2003), it can be speculated that possible trans- interactions between GlialCAM molecules could also occur through these domains.

In the brain, *GLIALCAM* expression has been studied in mouse and humans by RT-PCR (Favre-Kontula et al., 2008; Spiegel et al., 2006), through a *LacZ* knock-in heterozygous mice (Favre-Kontula et al., 2008), and immunostainings in tissue or different primary cell cultures (Favre-Kontula et al., 2008; Lopez-Hernandez et al., 2011a). Altogether, these studies demonstrated that GlialCAM is mostly expressed in oligodendrocytes, ependymal cells, Bergmann glia and astrocytes. It is important to note here that expression of GlialCAM in astrocytes could not be detected by LacZ, as each method has a different degree of sensitivity. RT-PCR and immunohistochemical stainings also detected a minor expression of GlialCAM in specific neurons. GlialCAM is expressed by astrocytes in areas of cell-cell contacts (Favre-Kontula et al., 2008; Lopez-Hernandez et al., 2011a), and by oligodendrocytes in cell processes (Favre-Kontula et al., 2008). Co-localization studies by immunohistochemistry and EM immunogold and in tissue culture between MLC1 and GlialCAM revealed that both proteins co-localize at astrocytic end-feet in astrocyte-astrocyte junctions (Lopez-Hernandez et al., 2011a) (Figure 2). In contrast, no co-localization was observed in oligodendrocytes and myelin (Lopez-Hernandez et al., 2011a), suggesting that GlialCAM is not obligatory associated with MLC1 and may work alone or in association with other molecules.

The direct interaction between GlialCAM and MLC1 and the partial co-localization in the brain led us to hypothesize that *GLIALCAM* could be a second gene affected in MLC patients. Sequencing the exons and surrounding intronic regions of *GLIALCAM* in MLC patients without linkage to the MLC1 locus revealed two mutated alleles of the gene in patients with the classical phenotype, and only one mutated allele in those with the MLC improving phenotype. Genetic studies with the parents of the affected patients revealed that the classical and the benign phenotype are inherited in an autosomal recessive and dominant manner, respectively. Therefore, the approach used combining biochemical and genetical methodologies were extremely useful to find a second MLC gene (Lopez-Hernandez et al., 2011a).

Other studies using yeast-two hybrid screenings showed that MLC1 interacts with the β1 subunit of the Na$^+$,K$^+$-ATPase pump (Brignone et al., 2011). This interaction was detected between the intracellular N-terminus of MLC1 and the extracellular domain of the β1 subunit. Affinity-chromatography using ouabain, an inhibitor of the α-subunit of the ATPase, detected co-purification of MLC1 and the β1 subunit in intracellular compartments, but not at the plasma membrane fraction (Brignone et al., 2011). Co-localization in astrocytes between both proteins was found also in intracellular compartments, together with proteins of the DGC complex (Brignone et al., 2011). Probably, this protein could have a regulatory trafficking role in the biology of intracellular MLC1.

## Glialcam and MLC1 Relationship

As mentioned before, there is a difference between the localization of MLC1 in cell-cell junctions in primary culture or tissue astrocytes, and the localization of MLC1 alone in transfected cells, where it can be detected at the plasma membrane (Figure 2). However, after co-expression of MLC1 with GlialCAM, both proteins are enriched in cell contacts (Lopez-Hernandez et al., 2011b) (Figure 2). Thus, GlialCAM is an escort molecule necessary to bring MLC1 to cell junctions. In addition, GlialCAM is able to stabilize MLC1 containing MLC-related mutations, suggesting that this interaction may be important for MLC1 endoplasmatic reticulum exit (Lopez-Hernandez et al., 2011b). However, additional studies may be needed to support this hypothesis. GlialCAM targeting is independent of MLC1, as suggested by the unaffected localizations of GlialCAM in a brain from an MLC patient or in cultures of astrocytes without MLC1 (Lopez-Hernandez et al., 2011b).

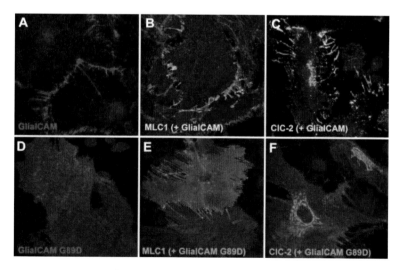

Figure 3. MLC-related mutations in GlialCAM abolish the targeting of GlialCAM, MLC1 and ClC-2 to astrocyte cell junctions. Localization in astrocyte junctions of GlialCAM (A), MLC1 (co-expressed with GlialCAM) (B) and ClC-2 (co-expressed with GlialCAM) (C) after adenoviral-mediated transduction. In contrast, the presence of a MLC-causing mutation (G89D) caused mislocalization of GlialCAM (D), MLC1 (E) or ClC-2 (F).

Most MLC-causing mutations in *GLIALCAM* seem to affect the traffic of GlialCAM to cell junctions (Figure 3), probably disrupting homophilic interactions between molecules in the same membrane (Lopez-Hernandez et al., 2011a; Lopez-Hernandez et al., 2011b). As GlialCAM is associated with MLC1, these mutations will also affect to the traffic of MLC1. From these studies it can be concluded that the localization of both proteins in cell junctions is key to carry on its physiological function. The molecular basis of the improving MLC phenotype and the classical phenotype by *GLIALCAM* mutations is also obscure, as both types of mutations seem to affect MLC1 protein trafficking. However, *GLIALCAM* dominant mutations also behave in a dominant manner in trafficking studies (Lopez-Hernandez et al., 2011a). Based on the localization of the dominant mutations in a putative pocket of the IgV domain, it was suggested that these mutations may affect trans-interactions with GlialCAM itself or with other unknown molecules (Lopez-Hernandez et al., 2011a).

## Glialcam Protein Network and the CLC-2 Chloride Channel

Motivated by the lack of co-localization between MLC1 and GlialCAM in oligodendrocytes, we searched for new GlialCAM-associated proteins (Jeworutzki et al., 2012). After affinity purification using two antibodies directed against GlialCAM, mass spectroscopy identified peptides corresponding to GlialCAM and MLC1, but also to the ClC-2 chloride channel. ClC-2 belongs to the ClC family of chloride channel/transport proteins (Jentsch et al., 2005), which form dimers and show a very complicate topology (Figure 1). What is the role of ClC-2 in the brain? In neurons expressing ClC-2, it is believed that the channel constitutes part of the background conductance regulating input resistance and provides an efflux pathway for chloride (Foldy et al., 2010; Rinke et al., 2010). The function of ClC-2 in glial cells is not clear, and it has been suggested to play a role in volume regulation or in the response to injuries (Ferroni et al., 1997; Makara et al., 2003; Zuniga et al., 2004). It is interesting to note that mice lacking ClC-2 exhibit a vacuolation of the white matter that resembles the pathology of MLC patients (Blanz et al., 2007). Furthermore, the vacuolation seems to depend on neuronal activity, as vacuoles were not observed in the optic nerve because the knockout mice are blind due to retinal degeneration (Blanz et al., 2007). Thus, based on the phenotype of the knockout mice, it has been suggested that ClC-2 may play a role in charge compensation during potassium influx or efflux by glial cells (Blanz et al., 2007). Furthermore, it was suggested that ClC-2 could potentially have a role in MLC pathogenesis. However, none of the patients without *MLC1* or *GLIALCAM* mutations carried mutations in *CLCN2* (Blanz et al., 2007; Scheper et al., 2010). Furthermore, MLC1 and ClC-2 could not be co-immunoprecipitated and deletion of MLC1 by RNA interference did not affect ClC-2 protein levels (Duarri et al., 2011). Hence, although very suggestive, the role of ClC-2 in MLC disease has not been established.

After the identification of ClC-2 as another binding partner of GlialCAM, we focused on the relationship between both proteins. Biochemical *in vitro* studies demonstrated that the interaction between GlialCAM and ClC-2 is direct (Jeworutzki et al., 2012). From a structural point of view, it is interesting to remark that two completely unrelated proteins (MLC1 and ClC-2) are able to interact with the same molecule. From the co-immunoprecipitation studies mentioned before, it was suggested that GlialCAM/MLC1 and GlialCAM/ClC-2 are independent complexes, although it can not be excluded that they could form higher order structures. As ClC proteins are present in all phylae (Jentsch et al., 2005), it was tested whether ClC-2 from *Drosophila melanogaster* (Flores et al., 2006), which do not express a GlialCAM ortholog, could still interact with GlialCAM. Interaction between both proteins was observed, suggesting that GlialCAM-ClC-2 interaction appeared later during evolution. GlialCAM was not found to interact with a typical ClC transporter such as ClC-5 (Picollo and Pusch, 2005; Scheel et al., 2005), and no interaction was observed between HepaCAM2 and ClC-2. Deletion of GlialCAM C-terminus or ClC-2 N-terminus (Grunder et al., 1992) did not abolish the interaction between both proteins. From these studies, and as ClC-2 is expressed in many tissues (Bosl et al., 2001; Thiemann et al., 1992), we concluded that GlialCAM is a brain specific auxiliary subunit of ClC-2 (Jeworutzki et al., 2012).

Which brain cells express both proteins? Double immunofluorescence experiments shown that both proteins co-localize in Bergmann glia, in astrocyte-astrocyte junctions at astrocytic endfeet around blood vessels (Sik et al., 2000) and in oligodendrocytes in myelinated fiber tracts (Jeworutzki et al Neuron, in revision). As both proteins were also present in astrocyte junctions, we tested whether GlialCAM changed the subcellular distribution of ClC-2 (Jeworutzki et al., 2012). In HeLa cells and astrocytes, GlialCAM was necessary to bring ClC-2 to cell junctions. In addition, as it happens with MLC1 and GlialCAM, MLC-related mutations in GlialCAM abolished the targeting of ClC-2 to junctions (Figure 3), pointing out to the fact that the localization of GlialCAM, ClC-2 and MLC1 in cell-cell junctions were indispensable for a correct physiological function.

As the function of ClC-2 can be measured by electrophysiology, we tested if GlialCAM could modify ClC-2-mediated currents. GlialCAM increased dramatically chloride currents, changing their properties of activation and its rectification, allowing more chloride flux at positive voltages (Jeworutzki et al., 2012). As the recorded activity of ClC-2 in brain slices or astrocytes have the appearance of ClC-2 alone (Ferroni et al., 1997; Makara et al., 2003; Nobile et al., 2000), we suggested that co-expression with GlialCAM may only be needed in special conditions, such as those that may occur during high neuronal activity, although evidence is lacking. MLC-related GlialCAM mutants do no affect to the activation of ClC-2 *in vitro*, hence further work is necessary to test whether influence ClC-2 function *in vivo*.

## Conclusion

Since the first MLC gene was discovered in 2001 (Leegwater et al., 2001), progress in the pathophysiological mechanisms of MLC disease has been hampered by the lack of knowledge of the function of the MLC1 protein. The study of cellular models of the disease has provided the first functional data that suggest that chloride currents are affected in MLC disease (Ridder et al., 2011). The collaboration between biochemistry and genetics was extremely useful to find the second disease gene (*GLIALCAM*) (Lopez-Hernandez et al., 2011a) and to clearly define the localization of MLC1 in cell-cell junctions (Duarri et al., 2011; Lopez-Hernandez et al., 2011b). Further biochemical studies have identified GlialCAM as the first auxiliary subunit of the ClC-2 chloride channel, potentially implicating ClC-2 in the pathology of the disease (Jeworutzki et al., 2012). New studies are needed to define the functional relationships and the physiological processes where these three proteins are involved. Studies with animal knockout models are in progress and, hopefully, they will provide new exciting clues about the pathology of MLC.

Although data are still preliminary, we hypothesized that MLC is a pathology that affects the process of potassium siphoning by glial cells. After high frequency firing of neurons, potassium is accumulated in the extracellular medium during the repolarization phase. Accumulation of potassium can cause unwanted neuronal depolarization, leading to neuronal hyperexcitability. Glial cells buffer this extracellular potassium, taking it out from the myelin and releasing it at blood vessels. This process implies a cellular pathway involving a network of glial cells connected by gap junctions, and implicating different ion channels and transporters (Kofuji and Newman, 2004). This pathway has to be extremely well regulated, as excessive buffering could lead to lack of excitability, and then, has to work as a directional pathway. Thus, disruption in mice of ion channels involved in this process lead to excitability alterations and vacuolation, due to accumulation of osmotically-driven water.

Ion and water handling in the brain is a very important process with high biomedical impact, as many human diseases are affected in this process, such as stroke, brain edema after head trauma or epilepsy (Amiry-Moghaddam and Ottersen, 2003). We believe that the study of MLC will provide new conceptual ideas about these diseases. Furthermore, the comprehension of the pathophysiology of MLC will speed up the development of new therapies for MLC patients, and perhaps to other alterations related with water homeostasis in the brain.

## Acknowledgments

We thank all members of the lab and to our collaborators for their support. I thank to Virginia Nunes for comments on the book chapter. Studies in our lab are supported by SAF 2009-07014, PS09/02672-ERARE, ELA Foundation 2009-017C4 project, 2009 SGR and an ICREA Academia prize.

## References

Ambrosini, E., Serafini, B., Lanciotti, A., Tosini, F., Scialpi, F., Psaila, R., Raggi, C., Di Girolamo, F., Petrucci, T. C., and Aloisi, F. (2008). Biochemical characterization of MLC1 protein in astrocytes and its association with the dystrophin-glycoprotein complex. *Mol. Cell. Neurosci.* 37, 480-493.

Amiry-Moghaddam, M., Frydenlund, D. S., and Ottersen, O. P. (2004). Anchoring of aquaporin-4 in brain: molecular mechanisms and implications for the physiology and pathophysiology of water transport. *Neuroscience* 129, 999-1010.

Amiry-Moghaddam, M., and Ottersen, O. P. (2003). The molecular basis of water transport in the brain. *Nat. Rev. Neurosci.* 4, 991-1001.

Amiry-Moghaddam, M., Williamson, A., Palomba, M., Eid, T., de Lanerolle, N. C., Nagelhus, E. A., Adams, M. E., Froehner, S. C., Agre, P., and Ottersen, O.P. (2003). Delayed K+ clearance associated with aquaporin-4 mislocalization: phenotypic defects in brains of alpha-syntrophin-null mice. *Proc. Natl. Acad. Sci. U.S.A.* 100, 13615-13620.

Attwell, D., Buchan, A. M., Charpak, S., Lauritzen, M., Macvicar, B. A., and Newman, E.A. (2010). Glial and neuronal control of brain blood flow. *Nature* 468, 232-243.

Becker, M., Matzner, M., and Gerisch, G. (1999). Drainin required for membrane fusion of the contractile vacuole in Dictyostelium is the prototype of a protein family also represented in man. *EMBO J.* 18, 3305-3316.

Blanz, J., Schweizer, M., Auberson, M., Maier, H., Muenscher, A., Hubner, C. A., and Jentsch, T. J. (2007). Leukoencephalopathy upon disruption of the chloride channel ClC-2. *J. Neurosci.* 27, 6581-6589.

Blattner, R., Von Moers, A., Leegwater, P. A., Hanefeld, F. A., Van Der Knaap, M.S., and Kohler, W. (2003). Clinical and genetic heterogeneity in megalencephalic leukoencephalopathy with subcortical cysts (MLC). *Neuropediatrics* 34, 215-218.

Boor, I., Nagtegaal, M., Kamphorst, W., van der Valk, P., Pronk, J. C., van Horssen, J., Dinopoulos, A., Bove, K. E., Pascual-Castroviejo, I., Muntoni, F., *et al.* (2007). MLC1 is associated with the dystrophin-glycoprotein complex at astrocytic endfeet. *Acta Neuropathol.* 114, 403-410.

Boor, P. K., de Groot, K., Waisfisz, Q., Kamphorst, W., Oudejans, C. B., Powers, J. M., Pronk, J. C., Scheper, G. C., and van der Knaap, M. S. (2005). MLC1: a novel protein in distal astroglial processes. *J. Neuropathol. Exp. Neurol.* 64, 412-419.

Bosl, M. R., Stein, V., Hubner, C., Zdebik, A. A., Jordt, S. E., Mukhopadhyay, A. K., Davidoff, M. S., Holstein, A. F., and Jentsch, T. J. (2001). Male germ cells and photoreceptors, both dependent on close cell-cell interactions, degenerate upon ClC-2 Cl(-) channel disruption. *EMBO J.* 20, 1289-1299.

Brignone, M. S., Lanciotti, A., Macioce, P., Macchia, G., Gaetani, M., Aloisi, F., Petrucci, T. C., and Ambrosini, E. (2011). The beta1 subunit of the Na,K-ATPase pump interacts with megalencephalic leucoencephalopathy with subcortical cysts protein 1 (MLC1) in brain astrocytes: new insights into MLC pathogenesis. *Hum. Mol. Genet.* 20, 90-103.

Chung Moh, M., Hoon Lee, L., and Shen, S. (2005). Cloning and characterization of hepaCAM, a novel Ig-like cell adhesion molecule suppressed in human hepatocellular carcinoma. *J. Hepatol.* 42, 833-841.

Devaney, J. M., Donarum, E. A., Brown, K. M., Meyer, J., Stober, G., Lesch, K. P., Nestadt, G., Stephan, D. A., and Pulver, A. E. (2002). No missense mutation of WKL1 in a subgroup of probands with schizophrenia. *Mol. Psychiatry* 7, 419-423.

Duarri, A., Lopez de Heredia, M., Capdevila-Nortes, X., Ridder, M. C., Montolio, M., Lopez-Hernandez, T., Boor, I., Lien, C. F., Hagemann, T., Messing, A., *et al.* (2011). Knockdown of MLC1 in primary astrocytes causes cell vacuolation: A MLC disease cell model. *Neurobiol. Dis.* 43, 228-238.

Duarri, A., Teijido, O., Lopez-Hernandez, T., Scheper, G. C., Barriere, H., Boor, I., Aguado, F., Zorzano, A., Palacin, M., Martinez, A. et al. (2008). Molecular pathogenesis of megalencephalic leukoencephalopathy with subcortical cysts: mutations in MLC1 cause folding defects. *Hum. Mol. Genet.* 17, 3728-3739.

Engel, P., Eck, M. J., and Terhorst, C. (2003). The SAP and SLAM families in immune responses and X-linked lymphoproliferative disease. *Nat. Rev. Immunol.* 3, 813-821.

Ernest, N. J., Weaver, A. K., Van Duyn, L. B., and Sontheimer, H. W. (2005). Relative contribution of chloride channels and transporters to regulatory volume decrease in human glioma cells. *Am. J. Physiol. Cell. Physiol.* 288, C1451-60.

Eroglu, C., and Barres, B.A. (2010). Regulation of synaptic connectivity by glia. *Nature* 468, 223-231.

Fanning, A. S., and Anderson, J. M. (2009). Zonula occludens-1 and -2 are cytosolic scaffolds that regulate the assembly of cellular junctions. *Ann. N. Y. Acad. Sci.* 1165, 113-120.

Favre-Kontula, L., Rolland, A., Bernasconi, L., Karmirantzou, M., Power, C., Antonsson, B., and Boschert, U. (2008). GlialCAM, an immunoglobulin-like cell adhesion molecule is expressed in glial cells of the central nervous system. *Glia* 56, 633-645.

Ferroni, S., Marchini, C., Nobile, M., and Rapisarda, C. (1997). Characterization of an inwardly rectifying chloride conductance expressed by cultured rat cortical astrocytes. *Glia* 21, 217-227.

Flores, C. A., Niemeyer, M. I., Sepulveda, F. V., and Cid, L. P. (2006). Two splice variants derived from a Drosophila melanogaster candidate ClC gene generate ClC-2-type Cl-channels. *Mol. Membr. Biol.* 23, 149-156.

Foldy, C., Lee, S. H., Morgan, R. J., and Soltesz, I. (2010). Regulation of fast-spiking basket cell synapses by the chloride channel ClC-2. *Nat. Neurosci.* 13, 1047-1049.

Gorospe, J. R., and Maletkovic, J. (2006). Alexander disease and megalencephalic leukoencephalopathy with subcortical cysts: leukodystrophies arising from astrocyte dysfunction. *Ment. Retard. Dev. Disabil. Res. Rev.* 12, 113-122.

Grunder, S., Thiemann, A., Pusch, M., and Jentsch, T. J. (1992). Regions involved in the opening of ClC-2 chloride channel by voltage and cell volume. *Nature* 360, 759-762.

Gurezka, R., Laage, R., Brosig, B., and Langosch, D. (1999). A heptad motif of leucine residues found in membrane proteins can drive self-assembly of artificial transmembrane segments. *J. Biol. Chem.* 274, 9265-9270.

Haj-Yasein, N. N., Jensen, V., Vindedal, G. F., Gundersen, G. A., Klungland, A., Ottersen, O. P., Hvalby, O., and Nagelhus, E.A. (2011). Evidence that compromised K(+) spatial buffering contributes to the epileptogenic effect of mutations in the human kir4.1 gene (KCNJ10). *Glia* 59, 1635-1642.

He, Y., Wu, X., Luo, C., Wang, L., and Lin, J. (2010). Functional significance of the hepaCAM gene in bladder cancer. *BMC Cancer* 10, 83.

Ilja Boor, P. K., de Groot, K., Mejaski-Bosnjak, V., Brenner, C., van der Knaap, M. S., Scheper, G. C., and Pronk, J. C. (2006). Megalencephalic leukoencephalopathy with subcortical cysts: an update and extended mutation analysis of MLC1. *Hum. Mutat.* 27, 505-512.

Jentsch, T. J., Poet, M., Fuhrmann, J. C., and Zdebik, A. A. (2005). Physiological functions of CLC Cl- channels gleaned from human genetic disease and mouse models. *Annu. Rev. Physiol.* 67, 779-807.

Jeworutzki E., López-Hernández T., Capdevila-Nortes X., Sirisi S., Bengtsson L., Montolio M., Zifarelli G., Arnedo T., Müller C.S., Schulte U., Nunes V., Martínez A., Jentsch T.J., Gasull X., Pusch M., Estévez R.. (2012). GlialCAM, a protein defective in a leukodystrophy, serves as a ClC-2 (Cl-) channel auxiliary subunit. *Neuron* 73, 951-961.

Kaganovich, M., Peretz, A., Ritsner, M., Bening Abu-Shach, U., Attali, B., and Navon, R. (2004). Is the WKL1 gene associated with schizophrenia? *Am. J. Med. Genet. B. Neuropsychiatr. Genet.* 125B, 31-37.

Kaye, E. M. (2001). Update on genetic disorders affecting white matter. *Pediatr. Neurol.* 24, 11-24.

Kimelberg, H. K. (2004). Increased release of excitatory amino acids by the actions of ATP and peroxynitrite on volume-regulated anion channels (VRACs) in astrocytes. *Neurochem. Int.* 45, 511-519.

Kofuji, P., and Newman, E. A. (2004). Potassium buffering in the central nervous system. *Neuroscience* 129, 1045-1056.

Krapivinsky, G. B., Ackerman, M. J., Gordon, E. A., Krapivinsky, L. D., and Clapham, D. E. (1994). Molecular characterization of a swelling-induced chloride conductance regulatory protein, pICln. *Cell* 76, 439-448.

Lanciotti, A., Brignone, M. S., Camerini, S., Serafini, B., Macchia, G., Raggi, C., Molinari, P., Crescenzi, M., Musumeci, M., Sargiacomo, M., *et al.* (2010). MLC1 trafficking and membrane expression in astrocytes: role of caveolin-1 and phosphorylation. *Neurobiol. Dis.* 37, 581-595.

Lee, L. H., Moh, M. C., Zhang, T., and Shen, S. (2009). The immunoglobulin-like cell adhesion molecule hepaCAM induces differentiation of human glioblastoma U373-MG cells. *J. Cell. Biochem.* 107, 1129-1138.

Leegwater, P. A., Boor, P. K., Pronk, J. C., and van der Knaap, M. S. (2002a). Association of WKL1/MLC1 with catatonic schizophrenia. *Mol. Psychiatry* 7, 1037; *author reply* 1037-8.

Leegwater, P. A., Boor, P. K., Yuan, B. Q., van der Steen, J., Visser, A., Konst, A. A., Oudejans, C. B., Schutgens, R. B., Pronk, J. C., and van der Knaap, M. S. (2002b). Identification of novel mutations in MLC1 responsible for megalencephalic leukoencephalopathy with subcortical cysts. *Hum. Genet.* 110, 279-283.

Leegwater, P. A., Yuan, B. Q., van der Steen, J., Mulders, J., Konst, A. A., Boor, P. K., Mejaski-Bosnjak, V., van der Maarel, S. M., Frants, R. R., Oudejans, C. B., *et al.* (2001). Mutations of MLC1 (KIAA0027), encoding a putative membrane protein, cause megalencephalic leukoencephalopathy with subcortical cysts. *Am. J. Hum. Genet.* 68, 831-838.

Lopez-Hernandez, T., Ridder, M. C., Montolio, M., Capdevila-Nortes, X., Polder, E., Sirisi, S., Duarri, A., Schulte, U., Fakler, B., Nunes, V., *et al.* (2011a). Mutant GlialCAM Causes Megalencephalic Leukoencephalopathy with Subcortical Cysts, Benign Familial Macrocephaly, and Macrocephaly with Retardation and Autism. *Am. J. Hum. Genet.* 88, 422-432.

Lopez-Hernandez, T., Sirisi, S., Capdevila-Nortes, X., Montolio, M., Fernandez-Duenas, V., Scheper, G. C., van der Knaap, M.S., Casquero, P., Ciruela, F., Ferrer, I., Nunes, V., and Estevez, R. (2011b). Molecular mechanisms of MLC1 and GLIALCAM mutations in megalencephalic leukoencephalopathy with subcortical cysts. *Hum. Mol. Genet.* 20, 3266-3277.

Makara, J. K., Rappert, A., Matthias, K., Steinhauser, C., Spat, A., and Kettenmann, H. (2003). Astrocytes from mouse brain slices express ClC-2-mediated Cl- currents regulated during development and after injury. *Mol. Cell. Neurosci.* 23, 521-530.

Mathiisen, T. M., Lehre, K. P., Danbolt, N. C., and Ottersen, O. P. (2010). The perivascular astroglial sheath provides a complete covering of the brain microvessels: an electron microscopic 3D reconstruction. *Glia* 58, 1094-1103.

Messing, A., and Brenner, M. (2003). GFAP: functional implications gleaned from studies of genetically engineered mice. *Glia* 43, 87-90.

Messing, A., Daniels, C. M., and Hagemann, T. L. (2010). Strategies for treatment in Alexander disease. *Neurotherapeutics* 7, 507-515.

Meyer, J., Huberth, A., Ortega, G., Syagailo, Y. V., Jatzke, S., Mossner, R., Strom, T. M., Ulzheimer-Teuber, I., Stober, G., Schmitt, A., and Lesch, K.P. (2001). A missense mutation in a novel gene encoding a putative cation channel is associated with catatonic schizophrenia in a large pedigree. *Mol. Psychiatry* 6, 302-306.

Moh, M. C., Lee, L. H., Zhang, T., and Shen, S. (2009a). Interaction of the immunoglobulin-like cell adhesion molecule hepaCAM with caveolin-1. *Biochem. Biophys. Res. Commun.* 378, 755-760.

Moh, M. C., Tian, Q., Zhang, T., Lee, L. H., and Shen, S. (2009b). The immunoglobulin-like cell adhesion molecule hepaCAM modulates cell adhesion and motility through direct interaction with the actin cytoskeleton. *J. Cell. Physiol.* 219, 382-391.

Moh, M. C., Zhang, C., Luo, C., Lee, L. H., and Shen, S. (2005). Structural and functional analyses of a novel ig-like cell adhesion molecule, hepaCAM, in the human breast carcinoma MCF7 cells. *J. Biol. Chem.* 280, 27366-27374.

Montagna, G., Teijido, O., Eymard-Pierre, E., Muraki, K., Cohen, B., Loizzo, A., Grosso, P., Tedeschi, G., Palacin, M., Boespflug-Tanguy, O., et al. (2006). Vacuolating megalencephalic leukoencephalopathy with subcortical cysts: functional studies of novel variants in MLC1. *Hum. Mutat.* 27, 292.

Nave, K. A. (2010). Myelination and support of axonal integrity by glia. *Nature* 468, 244-252.

Neusch, C., Rozengurt, N., Jacobs, R. E., Lester, H. A., and Kofuji, P. (2001). Kir4.1 potassium channel subunit is crucial for oligodendrocyte development and *in vivo* myelination. *J. Neurosci.* 21, 5429-5438.

Nobile, M., Pusch, M., Rapisarda, C., and Ferroni, S. (2000). Single-channel analysis of a ClC-2-like chloride conductance in cultured rat cortical astrocytes. *FEBS Lett.* 479, 10-14.

Pasantes-Morales, H., Lezama, R. A., Ramos-Mandujano, G., and Tuz, K. L. (2006). Mechanisms of cell volume regulation in hypo-osmolality. *Am. J. Med.* 119, S4-11.

Pascual-Castroviejo, I., van der Knaap, M. S., Pronk, J. C., Garcia-Segura, J. M., Gutierrez-Molina, M., and Pascual-Pascual, S. I. (2005). Vacuolating megalencephalic leukoencephalopathy: 24 year follow-up of two siblings. *Neurologia* 20, 33-40.

Patrono, C., Di Giacinto, G., Eymard-Pierre, E., Santorelli, F. M., Rodriguez, D., De Stefano, N., Federico, A., Gatti, R., Benigno, V., Megarbane, A., et al. (2003). Genetic heterogeneity of megalencephalic leukoencephalopathy and subcortical cysts. *Neurology* 61, 534-537.

Paulmichl, M., Li, Y., Wickman, K., Ackerman, M., Peralta, E., and Clapham, D. (1992). New mammalian chloride channel identified by expression cloning. *Nature* 356, 238-241.

Picollo, A., and Pusch, M. (2005). Chloride/proton antiporter activity of mammalian CLC proteins ClC-4 and ClC-5. *Nature* 436, 420-423.

Pineda, M., Fernandez, E., Torrents, D., Estevez, R., Lopez, C., Camps, M., Lloberas, J., Zorzano, A., and Palacin, M. (1999). Identification of a membrane protein, LAT-2, that Co-expresses with 4F2 heavy chain, an L-type amino acid transport activity with broad specificity for small and large zwitterionic amino acids. *J. Biol. Chem.* 274, 19738-19744.

Prust, M., Wang, J., Morizono, H., Messing, A., Brenner, M., Gordon, E., Hartka, T., Sokohl, A., Schiffmann, R., Gordish-Dressman, H., *et al.* (2011). GFAP mutations, age at onset, and clinical subtypes in Alexander disease. *Neurology.*

Pu, W. T., Krapivinsky, G. B., Krapivinsky, L., and Clapham, D. E. (1999). pICln inhibits snRNP biogenesis by binding core spliceosomal proteins. *Mol. Cell. Biol.* 19, 4113-4120.

Ridder M.C., Boor I., Lodder J.C., Postma N.L., Capdevila-Nortes X., Duarri A., Brussaard A.B., Estévez R., Scheper G.C., Mansvelder H.D., van der Knaap M.S. (2011). Megalencephalic leukoencephalopathy with cysts: defect in chloride currents and cell volume regulation. *Brain* 134, 3342-3354.

Rinke, I., Artmann, J., and Stein, V. (2010). ClC-2 voltage-gated channels constitute part of the background conductance and assist chloride extrusion. *J. Neurosci.* 30, 4776-4786.

Rubie, C., Lichtner, P., Gartner, J., Siekiera, M., Uziel, G., Kohlmann, B., Kohlschutter, A., Meitinger, T., Stober, G., and Bettecken, T. (2003). Sequence diversity of KIAA0027/MLC1: are megalencephalic leukoencephalopathy and schizophrenia allelic disorders? *Hum. Mutat.* 21, 45-52.

Scheel, O., Zdebik, A. A., Lourdel, S., and Jentsch, T. J. (2005). Voltage-dependent electrogenic chloride/proton exchange by endosomal CLC proteins. *Nature* 436, 424-427.

Scheper, G. C., van Berkel, C. G., Leisle, L., de Groot, K. E., Errami, A., Jentsch, T. J., and Van der Knaap, M. S. (2010). Analysis of CLCN2 as candidate gene for megalencephalic leukoencephalopathy with subcortical cysts. *Genet. Test. Mol. Biomarkers* 14, 255-257.

Schiffmann, R., and Boespflug-Tanguy, O. (2001). An update on the leukodsytrophies. *Curr. Opin. Neurol.* 14, 789-794.

Schiffmann, R., and van der Knaap, M. S. (2004). The latest on leukodystrophies. *Curr. Opin. Neurol.* 17, 187-192.

Schmitt, A., Gofferje, V., Weber, M., Meyer, J., Mossner, R., and Lesch, K. P. (2003). The brain-specific protein MLC1 implicated in megalencephalic leukoencephalopathy with subcortical cysts is expressed in glial cells in the murine brain. *Glia* 44, 283-295.

Selch, S., Strobel, A., Haderlein, J., Meyer, J., Jacob, C. P., Schmitt, A., Lesch, K. P., and Reif, A. (2007). MLC1 polymorphisms are specifically associated with periodic catatonia, a subgroup of chronic schizophrenia. *Biol. Psychiatry* 61, 1211-1214.

Sik, A., Smith, R. L., and Freund, T. F. (2000). Distribution of chloride channel-2-immunoreactive neuronal and astrocytic processes in the hippocampus. *Neuroscience* 101, 51-65.

Singhal, B. S., Gorospe, J. R., and Naidu, S. (2003). Megalencephalic leukoencephalopathy with subcortical cysts. *J. Child Neurol.* 18, 646-652.

Spiegel, I., Adamsky, K., Eisenbach, M., Eshed, Y., Spiegel, A., Mirsky, R., Scherer, S. S., and Peles, E. (2006). Identification of novel cell-adhesion molecules in peripheral nerves using a signal-sequence trap. *Neuron. Glia Biol.* 2, 27-38.

Teijido, O., Casaroli-Marano, R., Kharkovets, T., Aguado, F., Zorzano, A., Palacin, M., Soriano, E., Martinez, A., and Estevez, R. (2007). Expression patterns of MLC1 protein in the central and peripheral nervous systems. *Neurobiol. Dis.* 26, 532-545.

Teijido, O., Martinez, A., Pusch, M., Zorzano, A., Soriano, E., Del Rio, J. A., Palacin, M., and Estevez, R. (2004). Localization and functional analyses of the MLC1 protein involved in megalencephalic leukoencephalopathy with subcortical cysts. *Hum. Mol. Genet.* 13, 2581-2594.

Thiemann, A., Grunder, S., Pusch, M., and Jentsch, T. J. (1992). A chloride channel widely expressed in epithelial and non-epithelial cells. *Nature* 356, 57-60.

Topcu, M., Gartioux, C., Ribierre, F., Yalcinkaya, C., Tokus, E., Oztekin, N., Beckmann, J. S., Ozguc, M., and Seboun, E. (2000). Vacuoliting megalencephalic leukoencephalopathy with subcortical cysts, mapped to chromosome 22qtel. *Am. J. Hum. Genet.* 66, 733-739.

Topcu, M., Saatci, I., Topcuoglu, M. A., Kose, G., and Kunak, B. (1998). Megalencephaly and leukodystrophy with mild clinical course: a report on 12 new cases. *Brain Dev.* 20, 142-153.

van der Knaap, M. S., Barth, P. G., Stroink, H., van Nieuwenhuizen, O., Arts, W. F., Hoogenraad, F., and Valk, J. (1995). Leukoencephalopathy with swelling and a discrepantly mild clinical course in eight children. *Ann. Neurol.* 37, 324-334.

van der Knaap, M. S., Barth, P. G., Vrensen, G. F., and Valk, J. (1996). Histopathology of an infantile-onset spongiform leukoencephalopathy with a discrepantly mild clinical course. *Acta Neuropathol.* 92, 206-212.

van der Knaap, M. S., Lai, V., Kohler, W., Salih, M. A., Fonseca, M. J., Benke, T. A., Wilson, C., Jayakar, P., Aine, M. R., Dom, L., et al. (2010). Megalencephalic leukoencephalopathy with cysts without MLC1 defect. *Ann. Neurol.* 67, 834-837.

van der Knaap, M. S., Valk, J., Barth, P. G., Smit, L. M., van Engelen, B. G., and Tortori Donati, P. (1995). Leukoencephalopathy with swelling in children and adolescents: MRI patterns and differential diagnosis. *Neuroradiology* 37, 679-686.

Verma, R., Mukerji, M., Grover, D., B-Rao, C., Das, S. K., Kubendran, S., Jain, S., and Brahmachari, S. K. (2005). MLC1 gene is associated with schizophrenia and bipolar disorder in Southern India. *Biol. Psychiatry* 58, 16-22.

Wang, J., Shang, J., Wu, Y., Gu, Q., Xiong, H., Ding, C., Wang, L., Gao, Z., Wu, X., and Jiang, Y. (2011). Identification of novel MLC1 mutations in Chinese patients with megalencephalic leukoencephalopathy with subcortical cysts (MLC). *J. Hum. Genet.* 56, 138-142.

Xun, C., Luo, C., Wu, X., Zhang, Q., Yan, L., and Shen, S. (2010). Expression of hepaCAM and its effect on proliferation of tumor cells in renal cell carcinoma. *Urology* 75, 828-834.

Yuzbasioglu, A., Topcu, M., Cetin Kocaefe, Y., and Ozguc, M. (2011). Novel mutations of the MLC1 gene in Turkish patients. *Eur. J. Med. Genet.* 54, 281-283.

Zhang, T., Moh, M. C., Lee, L. H., and Shen, S. (2010). The immunoglobulin-like cell adhesion molecule hepaCAM is cleaved in the human breast carcinoma MCF7 cells. *Int. J. Oncol.* 37, 155-165.

Zuniga, L., Niemeyer, M. I., Varela, D., Catalan, M., Cid, L. P., and Sepulveda, F.V. (2004). The voltage-dependent ClC-2 chloride channel has a dual gating mechanism. *J. Physiol.* 555, 671-682.

# Index

## #

10q23, 41

## A

accounting, 2
acetaminophen, 6
acid, ix, 1, 5, 6, 7, 9, 11, 12, 14, 19, 25, 26, 31, 32, 33, 42, 113, 121, 126, 128
acidic, 3, 12, 23, 53, 55, 62, 66, 68, 85, 118, 119
acidosis, 29
action potential, 4, 19, 38
acute myeloid leukemia, 50
adaptations, 85
adenosine, 2, 19, 39
adhesion(s), 115, 118, 125, 132, 134, 139, 140, 141, 142, 143, 144
adolescents, 144
adulthood, x, 65, 66
age, 72, 83, 92, 93, 94, 98, 101, 104, 105, 106, 110, 128, 143
aggregation, 133
aging process, 96
agonist, 46
alcohol abuse, 6
alcoholics, 6, 13, 14
allele, 134
alters, 35, 105
amino, 8, 13, 19, 37, 42, 45, 117, 128, 141, 143
amoeboid, 3
amphibia, 20, 33, 34
amplitude, 21, 28, 39
amyloid deposits, 23
amyotrophic lateral sclerosis, 23, 32, 77
analgesic, 13
anatomy, 104
anchoring, 23, 72
anesthetics, 20
ANOVA, 94, 95, 98, 100
antibody, 44, 120
anticancer drug, 10
antigen, 105, 109, 110, 115, 117, 119, 123
antigen-presenting cell(s), 109, 110, 115, 119
APC, 115
apoptosis, 38, 40, 54, 117
Argentina, 109
arrest, 24, 54
arterioles, 12
artery, 28, 29
arthropods, 111
aseptic, 111
aseptic meningitis, 111
astrocytic functions, ix, 18, 30
astrocytoma, 24, 26, 31, 45, 46, 49
astrogliosis, 4, 24, 29, 34, 109, 113, 114, 116, 117, 118, 123, 124
asymptomatic, 110
ataxia, 26, 30, 34, 127
ATP, 2, 19, 39, 141
attachment, 68, 124
autism, 128
autopsy, 83
autosomal recessive, 134
avian, 58
axons, xi, 2, 71, 72, 76, 127

## B

bacteria, 129
barium, 21
basal lamina, 72, 73, 75, 87, 131
base, 73, 84
basement membrane, 72
BBB, 109, 113, 114, 115, 116, 117

behavioral assessment, 91
behaviors, 86
beneficial effect, 9, 11
benign, 128, 134
biochemistry, 16, 51, 137
biomarkers, 102
biopsy, 127, 133
biosynthesis, 7, 51
bipolar disorder, 144
bladder cancer, 140
blood, ix, 1, 2, 4, 5, 11, 13, 18, 21, 26, 38, 39, 56, 57, 65, 69, 71, 72, 73, 75, 80, 109, 130, 132, 137, 138, 139
blood vessels, 2, 21, 56, 57, 65, 69, 71, 72, 73, 75, 80, 137, 138
blood-brain barrier, 1, 2, 4, 5, 11, 26
blood–brain-barrier component, ix
boutons, 107
brain functions, 21, 25, 56, 92, 39, 110, 126
branching, 86, 92, 96, 99
Brazil, 91
breast carcinoma, 142, 144

# C

$Ca^{2+}$, 18, 24, 31, 50, 124
calcium, 12, 15, 23, 38, 39, 42, 46, 47, 48, 50, 51, 120
cancer, x, 10, 24, 33, 75
carbohydrate, 53, 56
carbon, 38
cardiovascular disease(s), 13,14
cartilage, 44
catabolism, 112, 123
catalytic activity, 12
catatonia, 143
catatonic, 128, 141, 142
catatonic schizophrenia, 128, 141, 142
cation, 142
CD8+, 115, 116
cDNA, 12
cell body, 43, 71, 72, 76, 80, 134
cell cycle, 33, 40, 45, 54, 67, 79
cell death, 110, 113, 123
cell differentiation, 34, 71, 132
cell line(s), 24, 31, 44, 51, 132, 133
cell organization, 55, 56
central nervous system (CNS), xi, 1, 9, 14, 15, 18, 30, 31, 32, 33, 34, 47, 62, 66, 84, 85, 86, 109, 118, 119, 120, 121, 122, 123, 126, 127, 140, 141
centriole, 70, 72, 73, 75, 79
cerebellum, 5, 6, 7, 34, 50, 131
cerebral blood flow, 11, 49

cerebral cortex, 9, 31, 33, 34, 85
cerebral regulation of blood flow, ix
cerebrospinal fluid, 75, 84, 112, 120
challenges, 113
channel blocker, 21
chaperones, 130
chemical(s), 2, 3, 56, 130
chemokines, xi, 109, 110, 115, 118
children, 122, 144
choline, 103, 107
chondroitin sulfate, 117
choriomeningitis, 111, 112, 119, 121
chromatography, 135
chromosome, 127, 144
cilia, 70, 71, 72, 73, 75, 78, 84, 88
cilium, 56, 66, 67, 70, 71, 72, 75, 76, 79, 80, 83, 84
classification, 80
clinical syndrome, 128
clinical trials, 10
cloning, 12, 142
closure, 85
clustering, 24
clusters, 69, 73, 75, 76, 80
CNS, 1, 5, 14, 17, 18, 19, 22, 23, 26, 27, 28, 29, 34, 59, 60, 62, 66, 67, 104, 109, 110, 111, 112, 113, 114, 115, 117, 118, 119, 120, 121, 122, 123, 124, 125
cognitive development, 78, 92, 93, 101, 112
collaboration, 137
collateral, 48
color, 95, 98
communication, 15, 18, 38, 39, 48
compensation, 136
complexity, 107, 127
complications, xi, 110, 112, 122
composition, ix, x, 60, 62, 69, 77, 81, 82, 86, 87, 126
compounds, 5, 132
comprehension, 138
condensation, 83
conductance, 19, 20, 23, 28, 29, 31, 33, 36, 136, 140, 141, 142, 143
conduction, 19
conductor, 87
connectivity, 140
consolidation, 102
constituents, 5
consumption, 12, 39, 49
contractile vacuole, 139
controversial, 21, 39, 109, 116
convention, 5
cooperation, 22
*Copyright*, 57, 58
coronavirus, 113, 123

corpus callosum, 56, 68
correlation(s), 35, 98, 100, 103, 117
cortex, 5, 21, 26, 29, 30, 32, 44, 49, 50, 58, 68, 105, 107
cortical neurons, 119
costimulatory molecules, 123, 124
culture, 3, 7, 26, 75, 123, 130, 132, 134, 135
culture conditions, 3
cure, 10
CXC, 56
cyclooxygenase, ix, 1, 6, 7, 117
cysteine, 117
cytoarchitecture, 62, 69, 75, 86, 87
cytochrome(s), ix, 1, 2, 4, 5, 6, 7, 8, 9, 11, 12, 13, 14, 15
cytochrome p450, 6, 13
cytokines, xi, 46, 104, 109, 110, 113, 114, 115, 117, 118, 120, 121, 122
cytokinesis, 41
cytomegalovirus, 110, 111, 121
cytoplasm, 42, 44, 45, 46, 47, 67, 70, 71, 72, 73, 74, 75, 76, 78, 79, 80, 81, 82, 83, 84, 132
cytosine, 55
cytoskeleton, 40, 113, 132, 142
Czech Republic, 17

diffusion, 32
diffusivity, 30
dimerization, 43
direct action, 115
disability, 11
discharges, 20
discrimination, 53, 54, 60, 98
disease gene, 137
disease progression, 23, 30, 138
diseases, 4, 9, 11, 23, 29, 40, 66, 84, 110, 113, 127, 138
disorder, 25, 112, 125
distribution, xi, 5, 9, 22, 33, 34, 44, 45, 47, 49, 51, 80, 85, 91, 92, 93, 100, 103, 117, 132, 137
diversity, 11, 143
DNA, 41
doctors, 127
dogs, 68
domain structure, 37, 42
dorsolateral prefrontal cortex, 50
down-regulation, x, 24, 25, 27, 28, 29
Drosophila, 137, 140
drug metabolism, 4, 13
drugs, ix, 2, 5, 6, 10, 11, 14, 32
D-serine, 38, 48, 105, 106
dysplasia, 30

# D

damages, xi, 110
data set, 83
decay, 21
defects, 30, 139
degenerate, 139
degradation, 1, 11, 41, 83, 130
Delta, 111
dementia, 87
demyelinating disease, 117, 122, 124
dendrites, 78, 107
dendritic cell, 115, 118
dendrogram, 98
depolarization, 17, 20, 22, 25, 27, 28, 31, 138
deposition, 23, 85
deposits, 23
depressants, 6
depression, 20, 22, 30, 32, 35, 48, 118
derivatives, 38, 41
destruction, 110
detectable, 132
detection, 8, 38, 39, 44, 128, 131, 133
detoxification, 9, 10, 113
developing brain, 58
diacylglycerol, 50
differential diagnosis, 144

# E

EAE, 116
edema, 138
electrolyte, 34
electron, 3, 71, 83, 85, 142
electron microscopy, 71, 83
elongation, 86
embryogenesis, 62, 87
encephalitis, 109, 110, 111, 112, 117, 119, 120, 121, 123, 124
encephalomyelitis, 112, 120, 121, 122, 124
encoding, 26, 88, 103, 141, 142
endothelial cells, 11, 15, 44, 68, 80, 120
endothelium, 5, 114, 131
energy, ix, 1, 4, 12, 32, 39, 49, 127
environment, xi, 69, 92, 93, 94, 95, 96, 97, 98, 99, 100, 101, 102, 103, 105, 115
environmental change, 38, 93, 98
environmental conditions, 92, 102, 103, 107
environments, xi, 5, 91, 92, 93, 94, 102, 103, 106
enzyme(s), 1, 2, 4, 5, 6, 7, 8, 9, 10, 11, 14, 37, 40, 41, 42, 43, 44, 46, 47, 49, 114, 117
ependymal, 2, 56, 57, 62, 66, 68, 69, 70, 71, 72, 73, 74, 75, 78, 87, 131, 134

ependymal cell, 2, 56, 57, 62, 66, 68, 69, 70, 71, 72, 73, 75, 78, 87, 131, 134
epidemiology, 121
epilepsy, x, 17, 23, 25, 26, 35, 75, 138
epileptogenesis, 25
episodic memory, 100
epithelial cells, 75, 144
epitopes, 68, 123
epoxide hydroxylase, ix
Epstein-Barr virus, 110
equilibrium, 19
ethanol, 6, 12, 13, 15
etiology, ix
euchromatin, 73, 75, 80
evidence, ix, x, 4, 28, 29, 33, 53, 54, 55, 63, 66, 78, 84, 87, 102, 113, 116, 137
evolution, 84, 85, 127, 128, 137
excitability, 15, 19, 20, 25, 39, 48, 138
excitotoxicity, 34, 117
excretion, 10
exocytosis, 94, 102, 105
exons, 134
experimental autoimmune encephalomyelitis, 116, 124
experimental design, 95
exposure, 28, 29, 92, 110
extracellular matrix, 42, 56, 71, 72, 114, 116
extracellular space, ix, 18, 22, 35, 79, 81
extracts, 24
extrusion, 20, 143

# F

families, 37, 42, 43, 110, 111, 139
family members, 5, 6
fatty acids, 2, 7, 9, 38
fertilization, 40
fetus, 85
fiber, 2, 48, 68, 78, 102, 137
fibroblast growth factor, 60, 104
filament, 3, 68, 77, 83, 121
fine tuning, 47
fixation, 77, 83
fluid, 25, 28, 34, 35, 67, 126
fluorescence, 44
fMRI, 38
forebrain, 54, 55, 60, 61, 62, 63, 73, 75, 85, 86, 88, 116, 121
formation, 28, 46, 85, 91, 101, 113, 117, 120, 123, 134
free radicals, 116
frontal cortex, 7
functional architecture, 14, 33

functional changes, 26, 91, 101
funds, 103
fusion, 71, 74, 79, 129, 139

# G

GABA, 88, 92, 107, 114
GEF, 43
gender effects, 106
gene expression, 41, 48, 115, 121, 124
gene promoter, 58, 123
gene transfer, 60
genes, x, xi, 10, 21, 24, 35, 40, 41, 42, 45, 46, 115, 125, 126, 127
genetic disease, 110, 125, 127, 128, 30, 140, 141
genetics, 14, 16, 137
genome, 58, 112
germ cells, 139
glia, x, 12, 18, 20, 21, 24, 25, 28, 30, 31, 32, 34, 37, 40, 48, 54, 59, 60, 61, 63, 65, 67, 68, 72, 85, 87, 105, 117, 118, 120, 122, 134, 137, 140, 142
glial cells, x, xi, 2, 5, 8, 12, 21, 23, 28, 30, 32, 33, 34, 35, 38, 48, 51, 54, 55, 58, 62, 65, 67, 85, 86, 87, 89, 93, 102, 123, 126, 131, 136, 138, 140, 143
glioblastoma, 131, 141
glioma, 24, 34, 61, 140
glucose, 39, 49, 114
glue, 15, 48
glutamate, x, 2, 12, 14, 17, 18, 22, 23, 25, 27, 29, 31, 32, 33, 34, 35, 38, 39, 48, 68, 79, 92, 94, 102, 106, 107, 112, 114, 116, 118, 120, 123
glutamine, 4, 14, 34, 117, 120
glutathione, 117, 129
glycogen, ix, 12, 85
glycolysis, 39, 49
glycosylation, 128
grants, 59, 118
granules, 71, 78, 80
gray matter, ix, 33
group variance, 98
growth, xi, 7, 24, 40, 42, 48, 50, 55, 56, 57, 58, 59, 60, 72, 86, 113, 114, 116, 134
growth factor, 7, 42, 48, 55, 56, 57, 58, 59, 60, 72, 86, 113, 114, 116
GTPases, 43
guanine, 43
guidance, xi, 113

# H

head injury, 25
head trauma, 138

health, 1, 13
heart disease, 10
hepatic encephalopathy, 23, 34
hepatitis, 113, 123
hepatocellular carcinoma, 139
hepatoma, 51
herpes, 111, 121
herpesviruses, 109, 110
heterochromatin, 73, 75, 80, 83
heterogeneity, 11, 18, 34, 71, 104, 113, 124, 128, 139, 142
hippocampal astrocytes, xi, 6, 11, 15, 20, 25, 26, 28, 31, 48, 93
hippocampus, x, xi, 6, 7, 22, 25, 26, 28, 29, 30, 31, 32, 33, 34, 35, 39, 54, 62, 65, 66, 67, 68, 78, 81, 82, 83, 84, 86, 88, 89, 91, 101, 102, 103, 104, 105, 107, 143
histocompatibility antigens, 120
histogenesis, 85
history, 15, 93
HIV, 111, 112, 117, 118, 119, 121, 122
HIV-1, 112, 117, 118, 119, 122
homeostasis, x, xi, 2, 4, 17, 18, 20, 23, 25, 26, 27, 28, 29, 31, 33, 42, 125, 126, 127, 138
hormone(s), 17, 40, 42
hormone levels, 17
host, 75, 110, 112, 116, 118
housing, xi
HTLV, 111, 112, 121
human brain, x, 3, 5, 6, 7, 9, 14, 24, 35, 62, 86, 88, 115
human genome, 128
human immunodeficiency virus, 112, 122, 124
human subjects, 49
hybrid, 135
hydrolysis, 9, 46
hyperactivity, 20
hyperplasia, 98, 100, 102
hypertension, 12
hypertrophy, 107, 113
hypothalamus, 66, 87
hypothesis, 20, 26, 37, 38, 45, 66, 85, 128, 132, 135
hypoxia, 7, 8, 13, 15, 29, 30, 32

# I

identification, 31, 41, 58, 71, 78, 83, 122, 136
identity, 54, 60, 66, 94, 128, 130
IFN, 113, 115, 118, 121, 123
IFN-β, 115
image(s), 67, 70, 74, 76, 79, 81, 82, 126
immune function, 113
immune response, xi, 109, 110, 115, 117, 139
immunocompromised, 110, 111
immunofluorescence, 83, 133, 137
immunoglobulin, 133, 140, 141, 142, 144
immunohistochemistry, 23, 24, 131, 134
immunoprecipitation, 128, 131, 132, 133, 136
immunoreactivity, x, 24, 26, 32, 45, 50, 104, 120, 121
impairments, 101, 102, 103
improvements, 92, 93, 103
impulses, 34
in situ hybridization, 131
in vitro, x, 9, 10, 15, 26, 33, 46, 53, 54, 55, 58, 59, 75, 112, 118, 136, 137
in vivo, x, 7, 8, 10, 22, 28, 29, 30, 33, 39, 53, 54, 55, 58, 59, 106, 112, 116, 118, 122, 130, 132, 137, 142
India, 144
indirect effect, 117
individuals, 10, 101, 102, 127
induction, xi, 5, 13, 40, 105, 109, 113, 115
infection, xi, 109, 110, 111, 112, 113, 115, 116, 117, 118, 121, 122, 123, 124
infectious agents, 110
infectious mononucleosis, 110
inflammation, x, 9, 11, 14, 15, 29, 37, 46, 47, 48, 110, 119
inflammatory cells, 115
inflammatory disease, 109
inflammatory mediators, 117
inflammatory responses, 10
inheritance, 127
inhibition, 10, 11, 13, 22, 31, 116, 120
inhibitor, 10, 14, 15, 29, 45, 47, 124, 135
initiation, 122
injury(s), 1, 4, 7, 8, 10, 13, 15, 18, 23, 25, 26, 28, 29, 33, 34, 35, 104, 107, 109, 110, 113, 114, 116, 118, 121, 124, 127, 136, 141
inositol, x, 40, 41, 50
insects, 111
insertion, 43
integration, 39, 88
integrators, 39
integrity, 114, 142
interface, 5, 72, 77
interference, 132, 136
interferon (IFN), 115, 122, 123, 124
interferon gamma, 124
interneurons, x, 53, 56, 57
intervention, 10, 30
intracellular calcium, 4, 38, 39, 46
ion channels, 18, 19, 20, 21, 22, 24, 114, 125, 129, 138
ions, 18, 19, 20, 21, 22

ipsilateral, 88
irrigation, 114
ischemia, x, 8, 15, 17, 18, 20, 23, 28, 29, 30, 31, 32, 33, 34, 35, 105, 120, 121, 124
isozyme(s), 5, 42, 50
Italy, 37, 109

## K

$K^+$, x, 15, 17, 18, 19, 20, 21, 22, 23, 24, 25, 26, 27, 28, 29, 30, 31, 32, 33, 34, 35, 114, 135, 139
keratinocytes, 44
kidney, 13, 19

## L

labeling, 58, 83
laminar, 91, 92, 93, 101, 105
latency, 39, 95
lateral sclerosis, 24
lead, 20, 24, 26, 28, 129, 138
learning, 78, 88, 92, 93, 94, 101, 102, 103, 104, 106, 107
learning behavior, 106
lesions, 32, 91, 101, 105, 118, 124
leucine, 128, 140
leukemia, 121, 122
leukocytes, 115
ligand, 115
light, 59, 61, 69, 70, 72, 73, 74, 75, 79, 80, 82, 83, 102
lipid metabolism, x
liver, 2, 4, 5, 8, 13, 34 22, 41, 45, 49, 51, 85, 129, 130, 132, 134, 135, 136, 137
locus, 127, 134
long-term memory, 107
low temperatures, 130
lumen, 56, 65, 67, 69, 71, 72, 75, 76
Luo, 140, 142, 144
lymphoblast, 132, 133
lymphocytes, 112, 115, 117
lymphoma, 121

## M

machinery, 38, 130
macrophages, 113, 115, 123
magnetic resonance, 38
magnitude, 39
major depression, 40
major histocompatibility complex, xi, 109, 110, 114
majority, 9
mammalian brain, x, 31, 53, 54, 55, 58, 60, 61, 84, 87
mammals, 59, 65, 66, 68, 73, 78, 128, 134
man, 139
manipulation, 92
mass, 136
matrix, 80, 82, 115, 117
matrix metalloproteinase, 115, 117
matter, 2, 21, 39, 53
measles, 122
measurement(s), 13, 19, 25
mechanical stress, 20
medical, 127
megalencephalic leukoencephalopathy, xi, 139, 140, 141, 142, 143, 144
membranes, 5, 20, 21, 22, 114, 130, 131
memory, 78, 88, 92, 93, 94, 95, 98, 100, 101, 102, 103, 104, 105, 106, 107
memory performance, 98
memory processes, 106
meningitis, 109, 110, 111, 112
mental illness, 40
mental retardation, 26, 34, 128
messenger RNA, 104
messengers, 42
metabolic changes, 71
metabolic intermediates, ix, 1
metabolic pathways, 47
metabolism, ix, 2, 5, 6, 7, 8, 9, 12, 15, 39, 40, 42, 48, 49
metabolites, ix, 1, 5, 6, 11, 12, 14, 32
metabolized, 6, 10
metabolizing, vii, 1, 2, 4, 5, 8, 10, 13
methodological procedures, 98
methodology, 133
Mexico, 53
$Mg^{2+}$, 19
MHC, 114, 115, 124
MHC class II molecules, 115
microcirculation, 39
microphotographs, 44
microscope, 44, 69, 85
microscopy, 7, 77, 82, 83, 131
migration, 13, 60, 61, 62, 63, 67, 68, 86, 87, 89, 113
mitochondria, 72, 73, 75, 77, 78, 80, 83
mitosis, 67, 72, 73, 86
MMP, 117
model system, 106, 112, 132
models, 15, 23, 26, 35, 91, 112, 137, 140
modifications, 105
modulation of synaptic transmission, ix, 18
molecular biology, 51

molecular weight, 128
molecules, 4, 37, 38, 42, 47, 110, 113, 114, 115, 116, 117, 118, 134, 136, 143
monolayer, 72, 73
morphogenesis, 86
morphology, 2, 3, 23, 30, 68, 69, 71, 72, 74, 91, 92, 93, 100, 106, 126
morphometric, 94, 96, 97, 101, 102
motif, 42, 140
motor behavior, 92
motor neuron disease, 87
MRI, 126, 127, 144
mRNA(s), 23, 24, 25, 29, 45, 46, 50, 131, 132, 133
multiple sclerosis, 118, 119, 121, 124
multipotent, 54, 55, 58, 60, 61, 88, 114, 119
mumps, 112, 122
mutagenesis, 128, 129
mutant, 26, 58
mutation(s), 24, 26, 30, 31, 34, 122, 125, 126, 127, 128, 130, 135, 136, 137, 139, 140, 141, 142, 143, 144
myelin, xi, 112, 125, 127, 128, 133, 134, 138
myelinating regulation, ix
myeloid cells, 124

# N

$Na^+$, 19, 20, 21, 22, 48, 135
necrosis, 113, 122
neocortex, 23, 25, 86, 87, 89
neonates, 111
neoplastic tissue, 45
nervous system, ix, xi, 1, 14, 18, 37, 38, 44, 48, 66, 67, 84, 106, 109, 120, 121, 122, 124, 127
neural network, 39
neuroblasts, x, 54, 56, 57, 66, 69, 71, 72, 75, 78, 80, 88
neurodegeneration, 12, 23, 37, 59, 112, 113, 117, 122, 123
neurodegenerative disorders, 24, 106
neurofibrillary tangles, 23
neurogenesis, 54, 56, 58, 60, 61, 62, 66, 67, 68, 78, 81, 82, 83, 84, 85, 86, 87, 88, 89, 92, 93, 105, 107, 114
neuroinflammation, xi
neuroleptics, 6
neurological disease, 84, 102, 112
neuronal apoptosis, 88
neuronal cells, 56, 115
neuroprotection, ix, 121
neuroscience, xi, 104, 105, 106
neurotransmission, 40, 105

neurotransmitter(s), ix, 1, 2, 17, 18, 38, 40, 42, 72, 106, 113
neurotrophic factors, 92
nicotine, 6, 13
Nile, 111, 112, 124
nitric oxide, 38, 47, 92, 103, 104, 105, 106, 114, 118, 120, 122, 123
nitric oxide synthase, 47, 104, 105, 122, 123
nitrosamines, 6
NMDA receptors, 39
NMR, 49
nodes, 3
North America, 105
nuclear membrane, 71, 72, 73, 74, 75, 79, 80
nuclei, 67, 69, 73, 74, 78, 83, 107
nucleic acid, ix, 10
nucleotides, 38
nucleus, x, 24, 37, 40, 45, 47, 48, 60, 67, 70, 71, 73, 74, 75, 80, 81, 84, 110
null, 30, 131, 139
nutrient, 3

# O

occlusion, 8, 28
old age, 105
oligodendrocytes, ix, x, xi, 2, 18, 33, 53, 54, 55, 58, 61, 65, 66, 68, 73, 75, 86, 111, 123, 127, 131, 134, 136, 137
oligomerization, 128
oligomers, 128
opioids, 6
optic nerve, 20, 136
optical microscopy, 83
organ, 50, 54, 114
organelle(s), 67, 71, 72, 73, 74, 76, 77, 78, 79, 80, 84
organize, 75
organs, 2, 13
osmolality, 142
osmotic stress, 35
overlap, 110
oxidation, 19
oxidative stress, 117
oxygen, 5, 32, 39

# P

pain, 9, 11
pancreas, 49
parallel, 48, 71, 74, 78, 80, 106
parallelism, 134
paralysis, 111

parenchyma, 56, 66, 69, 71, 72, 73, 110, 115, 116
parents, 134
participants, 116
pathogenesis, x, 18, 117, 120, 136, 139
pathology, 15, 23, 34, 50, 110, 122, 123, 126, 136, 137, 138
pathophysiological, 23, 25, 32, 101, 102, 103, 137
pathophysiology, xi, 28, 29, 51, 132, 138
pathways, ix, 1, 6, 7, 13, 33, 39, 46, 114, 117
pattern recognition, 110, 114
PCR, 24, 132, 134
PDGFR, 61
pedigree, 142
peptide(s), 9, 23, 32, 38, 46, 136
perinatal, 85
peripheral nervous system, 143
permeability, 17, 18, 20
permission, 57, 58
peroxynitrite, 141
personal communication, 132
PET, 38
pH, 4, 17, 19, 20, 23, 31
pharmaceutical, 10, 12
pharmacology, 16, 51
phenotype(s), 26, 45, 46, 92, 101, 102, 106, 125, 127, 128, 130, 134, 136
phenytoin, 15
phosphate(s), 9, 14, 40, 41
phospholipase C, x, 37, 40, 49, 50, 51
phospholipids, 15, 51
phosphorylation, 19, 42, 129, 141
photomicrographs, 3, 94
physical exercise, 92, 107
Physiological, 19, 20, 33, 125, 140
physiology, 1, 2, 34, 51, 106, 112, 138
plasma membrane, x, 5, 17, 24, 37, 41, 42, 73, 79, 80, 85, 129, 130, 132, 135
plasticity, ix, 48, 92, 93, 103, 104, 105, 106
platelets, 50
platform, 94, 95, 101, 102
polar, 42
polarity, 11, 40, 50, 85
polyamines, 19
polymerase, 24
polymerase chain reaction, 24
polymorphisms, 14, 143
polyunsaturated fat, ix, 1, 29
polyunsaturated fatty acids, 29
population, ix, 18, 54, 56, 59, 60, 101, 109
positron, 38
positron emission tomography, 38
potassium, x, 4, 17, 28, 30, 31, 32, 33, 34, 35, 36, 126, 128, 130, 136, 138, 142

precursor cells, 54, 55, 56, 60, 75, 83, 86
prefrontal cortex, 50
preservation, 77, 83
primary function, 19
primate, x, 73, 81, 83, 86, 87
probands, 139
producers, 116, 117
professionals, x, xi
progenitor cells, 55, 57, 62, 85, 86, 87, 113
progressive neurodegenerative disorder, 23
pro-inflammatory, 102
project, 75, 103, 138
proliferation, xi, 24, 28, 29, 30, 38, 45, 51, 55, 60, 61, 62, 66, 83, 85, 86, 88, 92, 112, 113, 119, 124, 132, 144
proline, 9, 134
promoter, 116
propagation, 38, 39
prostaglandins, 11
protease inhibitors, 114
proteasome, 130
protection, 7, 10, 102
protective role, 8, 117
protein family, 139
protein kinase C, 7, 15, 42, 129
proteinase, 51
proteins, ix, 2, 3, 4, 9, 10, 17, 19, 28, 29, 38, 40, 42, 43, 56, 68, 92, 113, 114, 117, 121, 126, 128, 129, 130, 131, 132, 133, 134, 135, 136, 137, 138, 140, 142, 143
proteoglycans, 72
proteolipid protein, 123
proto-oncogene, 114
prototype, 139
pulmonary hypertension, 14
purification, 133, 135, 136
purines, 38

# R

rabies virus, 112
reactivity, x
reagents, 131
reality, 84
receptors, xi, 4, 23, 37, 38, 39, 42, 43, 51, 103, 109, 110, 114, 117, 119, 122, 123
recognition, xi, 43, 91, 94, 95, 98, 100, 104
reconstruction, 97, 142
recovery, 110
rectification, 19, 137
recycling, 38
redistribution, 22
regenerate, 55

regeneration, 14, 84, 116, 117
regenerative capacity, 66
regression, 114
regulation of ion concentration, ix
renal cell carcinoma, 144
repair, ix, 31, 61, 114, 116, 120
replication, 41, 113, 117, 121
requirements, 39, 101
researchers, 20, 24, 40
residues, 8, 43, 128, 129, 134, 140
resistance, 28, 136
resolution, 13, 103
response, xi, 4, 5, 12, 18, 21, 23, 26, 28, 29, 37, 38, 40, 42, 61, 92, 102, 103, 104, 109, 110, 115, 116, 117, 118, 122, 123, 133, 136
restoration, 116
reticulum, 5, 42, 67, 71, 77, 78, 80, 130, 132, 135
retina, 17, 19, 21, 28, 32, 34, 49
retrovirus, 58, 112
retroviruses, 58, 109, 110, 112
rhabdoviruses, 109, 110
risk, 11
RNA, 120, 132, 136
RNAi, 33, 133
rodents, 9, 55, 56, 65, 66, 68, 71, 73, 74, 75, 78, 81, 83, 92

## S

SAP, 139
schizophrenia, 40, 50, 128, 139, 141, 143, 144
sclerosis, 25, 32, 35
secondary damage, 110
secretion, xi, 40, 49, 56, 109
segregation, 31
seizure, 22, 25, 26, 30, 32
selectivity, 19
self-assembly, 140
senescence, 102, 103, 106
sensitivity, 5, 19, 38, 39, 131, 134
sensors, 20
septum, 58, 72
serine, 42, 51, 129
serum, 55
shock, 114, 133
showing, 3, 8, 9, 11, 20, 22, 54, 67, 74, 79, 81, 82, 92, 116
siblings, 142
signal peptide, 133
signal transduction, 37, 40, 42, 46, 48
signalling, 48, 49
signals, 2, 38, 40, 48, 49, 56
signs, 118

smoking, 6
social interactions, 92
sodium, 4, 24, 33
solubility, 10
Spain, 54, 65, 125
spastic, 112
spasticity, 127
spatial cognition, 103
spatial information, 91, 101
spatial learning, 92, 93, 101, 104, 106
spatial memory, xi, 91, 92, 93, 94, 100, 101, 103, 104
specialization, 31
species, 18, 65, 66, 68, 92, 117
spectroscopy, 136
speech, 53
sperm, 51
spermatid, 44
spinal cord, 12, 23, 24, 26, 28, 32, 33, 34, 35, 66, 111, 112
spinal cord injury, 12, 28
sponge, 27
Sprague-Dawley rats, 14, 103
state(s), 1, 17, 18, 22, 23, 28
status epilepticus, 26, 32
stem cells, x, 18, 31, 53, 54, 55, 56, 57, 58, 59, 60, 61, 62, 65, 66, 67, 68, 73, 75, 79, 84, 86, 87, 88, 121
steroids, 38
sterols, 2
stimulation, 12, 20, 47, 49, 66, 92
stimulus, 21, 31, 39
storage, ix
strategic position, 115
stress, 5, 30, 88, 93, 104, 107, 118
striatum, 56, 58, 68
stroke, ix, 9, 10, 11, 15, 77, 88, 138
structure, xi, 1, 2, 9, 31, 40, 43, 121
subacute, 112
subarachnoidal, 22
subgranular zone (SGZ), x, 54, 65, 66, 78
substrate(s), 5, 6, 8, 9, 10, 13, 15, 39, 42
subventricular zone (SVZ), x, 53, 54, 57, 65, 66, 67, 68
suicide, 50
Sun, 35, 61
supplementation, 107
suppression, 47
survival, 51, 55, 115
swelling, 18, 29, 30, 118, 141, 144
symptoms, 109, 110, 112, 127
synapse, 13, 31, 38, 105
synaptic plasticity, 23, 39, 103, 107

synaptic strength, 48, 105
synaptic transmission, ix, 4, 18, 25, 38, 39, 113
synaptic vesicles, 88
syncytium, 18, 20, 21, 22, 29
syndrome, 26, 34, 50, 111
synthesis, 11, 42, 47, 115

# T

T cell(s), 116, 123, 124
T lymphocytes, 112, 123
target, xi, 4, 10, 12, 13, 14, 15, 30, 32, 42, 92, 101, 111
tau, 23
technical assistance, 59
techniques, 7
telencephalon, 62, 85, 86
temperature, 20
temporal lobe, 25, 26, 31, 35, 75
temporal lobe epilepsy, 25, 26, 31, 35
terminals, 39
TGF, 114, 117
T-helper cell, 115
therapeutic approaches, 30
therapeutic targets, 1, 13
therapy, 2, 66, 84, 127
three-dimensional reconstruction, 94, 97
threonine, 42
tissue, ix, x, 4, 10, 12, 17, 18, 20, 22, 23, 25, 26, 27, 28, 39, 40, 44, 55, 67, 78, 83, 120, 129, 130, 131, 132, 134, 135
tissue homeostasis, ix
TLR, 114
TLR2, 115, 123
TLR3, 115, 122, 123
TLR4, 115
TNF, 46, 112, 113, 117
TNF-α, 112, 113, 117
tobacco, 6
topology, 9, 12, 19, 134, 136
toxicity, ix, 117
toxicity depuration, ix
toys, 92
trafficking, 40, 115, 128, 135, 136, 141
training, 101, 106, 107
transcription, 8, 24, 40, 45, 46, 79
transduction, 37, 39, 40, 48, 51, 135
transfection, 24, 58, 133
transformation(s), 9, 45, 51, 86, 87, 113
transforming growth factor, 114
translation, 133
translocation, 42, 68
transmission, 38, 39, 80, 114, 120, 127
transport, 22, 23, 24, 33, 34, 35, 118, 128, 136, 138, 143
trauma, 23, 83, 124
treatment, ix, 10, 11, 15, 34, 45, 47, 49, 83, 127, 128, 132, 142
trial, 103
triggers, 113, 117, 119
tropism, 110, 119
tumor, x, 10, 24, 25, 30, 47, 112, 123, 144
tumor cells, 30, 144
tumor necrosis factor, 112, 123
tumor progression, x, 47
tumors, 24, 25, 35
tumours, 40, 134
turnover, 11
tyrosine, 43

# U

ubiquitin, 43
ultrastructure, 55, 66
underlying mechanisms, 11
uniform, 23
USA, 1, 12, 14, 15, 30, 34, 49, 51, 60, 61, 87, 88, 107, 119

# V

vaccine, 122
Valencia, xi, 65
variables, 94, 96, 98, 99, 105
variations, 10
vasculature, 68
vein, 44
velocity, 22
ventricle, 57, 65, 66, 67, 68, 69, 70, 71, 72, 73, 74, 75, 78
vertebrates, 68
vesicle, 71, 85
vessels, 21, 71, 72, 77
victims, 119
viral hemorrhagic fever, 112
viral infection, xi, 109, 110, 112, 113, 114, 115, 117, 118, 120, 122, 123
virus infection, 118, 119, 120, 121, 123, 124
viruses, xi, 109, 110, 111, 112, 115
visualization, 11
vulnerability, 120

## W

water, 22, 23, 29, 33, 35, 42, 93, 94, 98, 100, 101, 102, 104, 106, 126, 127, 130, 133, 138
wave propagation, 22
wealth, 1
Western blot, 24, 25, 128, 132
white matter, x, 2, 53, 54, 58, 125, 127, 136, 141
windows, 101
workers, x, xi
worldwide, 10, 11

## Y

Y-axis, 98, 100
yeast, 135
yield, 133
young adults, 101, 102

## Z

zinc, 9